NO MORE CAKES AND ALE?

*Dietary intelligence for gluten-free
adults and their food dudes*

SOPHIE NEWTON

TURNED BRAIN BOOKS

First published by Turned Brain Books in 2020

Copyright © Sophie Newton 2020

Sophie Newton asserts the moral right to be identified as the author of this work

The information in this book is not intended to replace the services of medical doctors, dietitians, or other healthcare professionals. For matters relating to your health, you should consult a medical doctor, and particularly in respect to any symptoms that may require diagnosis or medical attention. The author makes no representations or warranties with respect to any information offered or provided in this book regarding treatment, action, or the application of medication.

ISBN 978-1-8380262-1-9

Cover design by Dissect Designs

sophienewtonauthor.com

turnedbrainbooks.com

Contents

Introduction   1

Chapter 1: Preparing to go gluten-free   5

    The gluten-free diet in a nutshell   5

    What should happen before going gluten-free?   8

    What could happen after going gluten-free?   9

Chapter 2: Identifying and avoiding gluten   15

    The gluten roll: food and drink list   15

    A gluten dose by any other name   23

    A gluten dose by contamination   24

    A gluten dose put to the test   27

    The official language of gluten   28

Chapter 3: Understanding gluten-free nutrition   41

    Avoiding common mistakes   41

    Replacing the work of wheat   45

    Remedying common nutritional deficiencies   53

    Getting energised and repaired   59

    Supporting physical and mental health   74

    Oiling the wheels of nutritional savviness   79

Chapter 4: The lifelong gluten-free diet   87

    What to eat   87

    What not to eat   112

    When to eat   119

    How to eat   120

Meal planning   122

Rules of thumb for a balanced diet   124

Chapter 5: Lifehacks   128

Being prepared   128

Eating out   129

Eating at social and corporate events   133

Travelling   134

Wandering around on auto-pilot   136

Catering for the rest of the household   136

Getting food on prescription   137

Abandoning food on prescription   138

Helping an illiterate celiac   140

Going into hospital   140

Getting notified of product recalls   141

Dobbing in an incorrectly labelled product   142

Avoiding non-food sources of gluten   142

Eating out reprised   144

Other lifehacks   145

Chapter 6: What you don't need   146

You don't need a gluten-free recipe book   146

You don't need to go to a Free From show   150

You don't need teff flour   151

You don't need talk therapies   152

You don't need desperate marketing   153

Chapter 7: On the horizon   155

Drugs   155

Genetically modified wheat 156

Chapter 8: Cakes and ale and the good things in life 157

Recipes 160

Resources 170

Acknowledgements 176

About the author 177

Index 178

References 191

Introduction

This book is for you if you are an intelligent adult who (1) has celiac disease, non-celiac gluten sensitivity, wheat allergy, or dermatitis herpetiformis and thus must have a lifelong gluten-free diet, or (2) shops or cooks for another adult on a gluten-free diet, or (3) wants to go gluten-free for some other reason, for example, to attract a mate. (I wouldn't actually recommend the diet for the latter purpose because many people have an aversion to what they perceive as unwarranted fussiness about food. But it might work if the person you're trying to attract is gluten-free.)

You are a busy, down-to-earth person and do not want to spend your precious leisure time hanging out with others who have the same disease as you or seeing a therapist to emote about the meaning of your disease. You've got better things to do with your time, such as hiking, playing a sport, making music, going to concerts, reading, visiting friends, skating, learning a language, dancing, sailing, knitting, entering a cheese-rolling race, or creating sand sculptures. If you are going gluten-free for medical reasons, you already understand your diagnosis and now want to get on with the prescribed diet.

Enough about you. What about me? I was diagnosed with celiac disease as an adult. But don't worry; this is *not* a misery memoir.

Enough about both of us. What about this book? Some scientists and nutritionists have warned that going gluten-free may do more harm than good to health and that people who have no gluten-related disorder should not be encouraged to go gluten-free. Does this mean that this book encourages an unhealthy lifestyle? Hold on a minute. If a gluten-free diet can have adverse effects on "normal" people, surely it can also have adverse effects on people with gluten-related disorders — people who *must* have a gluten-free diet. We know that a gluten-free diet alleviates the symptoms of celiac disease and other gluten-related disorders. Do we have to accept that getting rid of the adverse effects of gluten entails accepting other problems? No, we don't. But it can happen. So listen up. What I am about to say is very important, and I shall say this only once — OK, no more than three or four times.

Simply eliminating wheat products (such as bread) from your diet or simply replacing them with gluten-free equivalents (such as gluten-free bread) would result in nutritional deficiencies, which would become more apparent over time.

The "eliminate" approach results in a reduced intake of vitamins, minerals, and fibre. The "replace with gluten-free equivalent" approach often provides equivalence only in terms of bulk and calories, and it also results in a reduced intake of nutrients, along with an increased intake of unhealthy ingredients. These approaches to gluten freedom are the basis for the warnings from the scientists. Happily, we will adopt a different approach.

Many sources of information about gluten-free diet just tell you what foods to avoid and then briefly say that this avoidance activity should form part of a balanced diet. There are two problems with this advice. First, it assumes that most people know what a balanced diet is. In reality, even people who try to eat well may base their food choices on randomly encountered information, which may be partial in both senses of the word. Second, people who do have a healthy diet may not know how to adapt it when instructed to go gluten-free because general guidelines on healthy eating typically recommend eating lots of whole-wheat products.

This book aims to provide all the information you need for a healthy, balanced gluten-free diet in one place. So you won't have to look in one place for a list of foods to avoid and another place for general guidance on healthy eating and then still have to figure out for yourself how to adapt the general guidance to the gluten-free requirement and how to put it all into practice.

The "one place" objective means that we'll cover some topics that are not specific to the gluten-free diet, such as cutting down on added sugars and processed food. Nonetheless, every section has been written with the needs of gluten-free people in mind. Whereas general books on nutrition mention the good sources of particular nutrients, this book mentions only the good *gluten-free* sources. I have gone beyond just removing wheat from common lists of foods because that could mean removing the food having the largest amount of a particular nutrient, leaving only foods with moderate or low amounts of it. In such cases, I have included some foods that you might not have previously eaten, such as quinoa. Similarly, the section on exercise contains not only general information on the relationship between calorie intake and calorie expenditure but also exercise tips specific to people with celiac disease, who have a higher risk of osteoporosis than the general population.

This is a diet book in the widest sense of the word "diet"; it is intended to equip you to select and prepare healthy gluten-free meals for the rest of your life rather than tell you exactly what to eat at every meal during a 14-day period. It will also help you to master the practicalities of gluten-free living, including shopping, understanding food labels, and eating out, all with minimum fuss. It is *not* a recipe book. However, it does contain tips on modifying ordinary recipes to make them gluten-free, and a few recipes are provided as examples.

If you're not actually interested in healthy eating and just want to do the minimum required to meet your doctor's instruction to go gluten free, you could just read the first two chapters and the "lifehacks" chapter. Then you will have enough information to avoid gluten-containing foods and gluten contamination, at home and when eating out. If you want recommendations for a healthy gluten-free diet but are not interested in the rationale for the recommendations, you could skip the chapter on understanding gluten-free nutrition. But if you've decided to use the need to go gluten-free as an opportunity to adopt a whole new healthy lifestyle, keep reading and continue until you get to the end!

A note for Brits: I have chosen to use the American English *celiac* spelling rather than the British English *coeliac*. There is a practical reason for getting used to the American spelling: searching the Web or medical databases for *celiac disease* yields much more information than searching for *coeliac disease*. If you enter *celiac disease* into the UK version of the search engine whose name is a famous misspelling of *googol*, you still get UK-specific results at the top.

Another note for Brits: This book assumes that the EU regulations on allergen labelling apply to the UK. Even if the British government were to relax the regulations for food sold in the UK, food manufacturers would probably continue to provide the allergen information demanded by the EU regulations; they already have processes in place to do so and they would otherwise lose sales at home and in Europe. Furthermore, enforcement of the EU labelling regulations in the UK is already done by the UK's own Food Standards Agency (FSA).

A note for non-Europeans: Most of this book is relevant to gluten-free people everywhere. Gluten is gluten worldwide. Moreover, in many countries, regulations governing the use of the term "gluten-free" are based on an international standard. I have tried to make this book relevant to an international audience, though there is a little bias toward Europe or the UK in some parts.

Chapter 1: Preparing to go gluten-free

The front page headline in *The Independent* newspaper on 6th April 2013 was "Britain running out of wheat as cold weather crisis hits farmers". Good news, I thought; the price of wheat will go up and food manufacturers and chefs will stop gratuitously adding it to dishes that did not traditionally have wheat in the recipe, making life easier for those of us on a gluten-free diet. My hopes that the food industry would find creative solutions to the impending shortage of an ingredient were dashed when I read the first sentence of the article: "Britain will be forced to become a net importer of wheat for the first time in a decade this year, after the recent bitter weather devastated crops."

For as long as vast quantities of wheat are grown or imported worldwide, you will be surrounded by gluten and you need to know how to avoid it while getting adequately nourished. So, what is the gluten-free diet?

The gluten-free diet in a nutshell

Gluten is a composite protein, comprising the proteins glutenin and gliadin. It is found in three cereal grains, namely, wheat, rye, and barley. Gluten is what makes dough elastic and cohesive. Indeed, the word "gluten" is related to the word "glue".

On a gluten-free diet, you cannot eat or drink anything containing wheat, rye, or barley. Consequently, there are hundreds of foods you may eat but only three you may not eat. How difficult can that be? If you buy fresh food and prepare it at home, it's easy. If you eat in restaurants, at social events, or in other people's homes or you get takeaway meals or pre-packed foods, it's difficult. In the EU, life got easier in December 2014, when the EU regulation on the provision of food information to consumers came into force. This regulation improved the rules on allergen labelling for pre-packed foods and introduced rules on information for loose foods. However, attitudes change more slowly than regulations. Therefore, it may take a while before all food businesses stick to both the letter and the spirit of this law. Furthermore, when you eat at friends' houses or at social events, you may find that the host is clueless about gluten. Consequently, you must become knowledgeable about what foods you can and cannot have.

Obviously, you have to avoid things containing flour ground from the grains of the three gluten-containing cereals — bread, cakes, biscuits, crackers, pasta, and so on. Equally obviously, you have to avoid things encased in pastry, such as pies. And things with a dough base, such as pizzas. Less obviously, you have to be aware that many soups, sauces, spreads, and pates are thickened with wheat flour, many frozen chips (French fries) are invisibly floured, the meat in many sausages and burgers is padded out with wheat, and some ice cream contains wheat. You also need to be aware that wheat has many guises — couscous, semolina, spelt, to name a few.

Many processed foods and restaurant meals contain gluten. Therefore, you must read the labels on processed foods and question servers when eating out.

Even with fresh food, you have to be careful. You may not, for example, eat salad sprinkled with croutons or doused in a gluten-containing dressing (as in some mustard dressings). You may not eat breaded ham or battered fish. And you may not eat meat or poultry that has been stuffed with a gluten-containing stuffing, marinated in a gluten-containing marinade, encased in pastry, dipped in a floury coating before frying, or covered in a gluten-containing sauce after serving.

Furthermore, if a meal contains a mixture of gluten-containing and gluten-free ingredients, you cannot eat just the gluten-free parts. For example, you cannot scrape the topping off a pizza or extract the filling from a sandwich or shake the sauce off a piece of meat because the topping or filling or meat is contaminated with gluten. For the same reason, you cannot eat food that has been fried in the same oil as gluten-containing food.

6

Contamination of naturally gluten-free foods with gluten is quite common. Oats are a particular concern due to the risk of contamination with gluten from other grains during harvesting or milling. You can have oats only if they are explicitly labelled as gluten-free. Contamination of other naturally gluten-free foods can occur further along the production process during manufacturing, packing, storage, or transportation. For example, many chocolate bars may contain gluten, even though they have no gluten-containing ingredients.

However, there are plenty of foods you may eat: meat, poultry, fish, shellfish, fruits, vegetables, legumes, eggs, milk, cheese, cream, yogurt, butter, cooking fats, oils, nuts, seeds, herbs, spices, and seaweed. You may also eat gluten-free cereals, including rice. And you may eat pseudo-cereals (non-cereal plants whose seeds are ground into flour), including quinoa, buckwheat, and amaranth. When making your own sauces or gravies, you can thicken them with cornflour (cornstarch) or arrowroot.

There is also plenty to drink: water, tea, coffee, herbal teas, most soft drinks (except barley water), milk, most milk-based drinks (but check the label on hot chocolate mixes), and most alcoholic drinks (except beer, unless it's special gluten-free beer).

You must consider everything that you ingest — not just food and drink but also any pills and potions you take. Almost all pharmaceutical products are gluten-free, but check the labels on complementary medicines and food supplements.

You may have any food or drink specifically labelled as gluten-free — unless subject to a product recall on the basis that gluten has been found in it.

You cannot simply eliminate wheat products or replace them with gluten-free equivalents because doing so would result in nutritional deficiencies, which would become more apparent over time. You need to replace the work of wheat in terms of its nutrition and its uses.

That's the diet in a nutshell. As it happens, a nutshell is the most reliable source of gluten-free food because the contents definitely cannot get contaminated on the way from the tree to your nut bowl.

What should happen before going gluten-free?

If your doctor suspects that you have celiac disease and wants to confirm the diagnosis with an endoscopy, you will be asked to continue eating gluten until the test has been done, to avoid a false negative result. During those couple of weeks, take the opportunity to have a few of your favourite gluten-containing foods one last time. For a retro experience, have a Farley's Rusk. It might well have been your first exposure to gluten and you can make it your last.

If you are going gluten-free for medical reasons, you should see a dietitian. In the UK, dietitians are the only health professionals who are qualified to provide information about special diets for medical conditions. (Nutritionists can provide information about food and healthy eating but not about special diets for medical conditions.)

In the UK, anyone who has been diagnosed with a condition requiring a gluten-free diet should get a referral to an NHS dietitian. You will probably be asked to keep a 4-day food diary before the appointment. If you cannot get an NHS consultation or you prefer to go private, search the database of the Freelance Dietitians Group (www.freelancedietitians.org) of the British Dietetic Association (www.bda.uk.com). If you find a dietitian another way, check that the person you have chosen is a Registered Dietitian by searching the register of the regulator, the Health & Care Professions Council (www.hpc-uk.org).

In other European countries, you can find the professional association for dietitians on the website of the European Federation of the Associations of Dietitians (www.efad.org).

For other countries, the International Confederation of Dietetic Associations lists the professional association on their website, www.internationaldietetics.org, if the association is a member.

A dietitian will review your current diet, give you information about the gluten-free diet, and give advice specific to your needs. This can be very useful. Even if you pride yourself on healthy eating habits, you may find that you have a blind spot with regard to a particular aspect of nutrition. Consulting a dietitian is especially important if you are combining the gluten-free diet with a special diet needed for another medical reason such as diabetes or a food allergy, or if you are vegetarian or vegan.

However, the initial appointment on the NHS is typically only 20 minutes and any follow-up appointments are also short, so there isn't time to cover the practicalities of everyday living on the gluten-free diet. In the rest of this book, I aim to do that.

What could happen after going gluten-free?

Before getting into the details of the gluten-free diet, let's get motivated to follow it by finding out what happens after you go gluten-free.

Shit happens, only better

If you have celiac disease and you had diarrhea or steatorrhea, your stools will become well-formed and your bowel movements will be better. If you had symptoms of malnutrition (for example, anemia due to malabsorption of iron) rather than digestive symptoms, you may nonetheless notice a change in your digestion and then realize that it hadn't been quite normal before. Digestive symptoms should improve noticeably within four weeks. You may well notice some positive changes within a couple of days.

Your health improves

If you have celiac disease, your gut will no longer be damaged by the autoimmune reaction to gluten. Thus it gradually heals and you absorb more of the nutrients in your food. Better nourishment obviously leads to better general health. Many people say that their hair, skin, and nails are in better condition after going gluten-free. Many report having more energy. You may even feel energetic enough to dance to the Bron-y-Aur Stomp.

Furthermore, the risks associated with untreated celiac disease, such as developing other autoimmune diseases or osteoporosis, will be reduced by sticking to the diet.

If you have gluten sensitivity or wheat allergy, sticking to the diet will eliminate your adverse reactions to wheat and thus improve your general sense of wellbeing.

Weighty things happen

Your weight could go either way. At the time of diagnosis, many celiacs are underweight due to malabsorption of nutrients. When absorption improves, you should put on weight. However, if you previously subsisted largely on gluten-containing foods and you just eliminate those from your diet without replacing them with other foods, you could lose weight. If you adopt a well-balanced gluten-free diet, there is a good chance that your weight will normalize and stay normal.

If you additionally adopt a well-balanced exercise regime, there's a good chance that your normal weight will comprise a normal proportion of muscle, bone, and fat.

If you're underweight and you gain weight, you may think that's good news. And you'd be right — up to a point. If you could previously eat any amount of food without getting fat, you risk getting fat while retaining an image of yourself as a slim person. To prevent this, weigh yourself every day so that it becomes a habit. Also monitor your waist measurement, aiming for it to be less than half your height. Ask a trusted friend to let you know if you start to get fat. Phone your friend today.

Some celiacs are somehow overweight at the time of diagnosis, as are some people with non-celiac gluten sensitivity or wheat allergy. Then there are overweight people without a medical condition who choose to go gluten-free in the hope that it will help with weight loss. Well, some overweight people lose weight on a gluten-free diet, whereas others get heavier. As with people who are underweight when they hit the gluten-free road, the outcome will depend largely on whether the new diet is well balanced.

You might get glutened

Unless you prepare all your own meals from scratch using only fresh ingredients, you will almost certainly accidentally ingest some gluten at some point. Unfortunately, this can happen even if you always read labels and always ask dinner party hosts and servers in restaurants for an explicit assurance that your meal is gluten-free. Someone somewhere will assure you that your meal is gluten-free when it isn't.

After going gluten-free, some people get an acute reaction when they ingest gluten. This is commonly called "getting glutened". The exact symptoms vary from person to person. Some people experience a return of previous symptoms. Some people experience different symptoms from those they had when they were chronically ill. Some people have an early warning system; within a few minutes of starting to eat something containing gluten, they feel unusual gurgling in the digestive system, presaging other symptoms. Some people experience a change in the symptoms of getting glutened after they have been gluten-free for a while.

There is an advantage to having noticeable reactions to gluten: it makes it easier to stick to the diet. Once you associate certain foods with feeling unwell, you simply won't want them. Having an early warning system is also useful — but only if you eat slowly. If your digestive system gurgles within a few minutes of starting to eat a meal but you have meanwhile gulped down the whole meal, it's of no use at all. So, if you are ever faced with food of uncertain gluten content, eat slowly. It's good to eat slowly, anyway.

Some people have asymptomatic celiac disease (formerly called silent celiac disease), in which blood tests are positive and an endoscopy shows intestinal damage but there are no symptoms when eating gluten. If you have been diagnosed with asymptomatic celiac disease, it is still important to stick to the diet, in order to avoid further silent damage and eventual symptomatic damage.

You might be tempted to make things worse

Being diagnosed with celiac disease is good news. I mean, it's not good to have the disease but if do you have it, it's good to be aware of it because then you can do something about it. Specifically, you can go gluten-free. This heals the intestinal damage and prevents further damage, thus improving your nutritional status. Consequently, a single dietary change resolves many symptoms. This is the cat's whiskers, the bee's knees, the ant's antennae. This is not the time to risk depriving yourself of some nutrients by unnecessarily taking on extra dietary restrictions. But this can happen if you mistake a normal variation in digestion for a gluten reaction or if you self-diagnose food allergies.

Everyone experiences variations in their digestion. Digestion may be affected by the time of day you eat, how much you eat, how often you eat, how fast you eat, whether you are stressed out when eating, and how much exercise you get. Although you need to take gluten reactions seriously, you also need to avoid a tendency to assume that every little change in your digestion is due to getting glutened.

Here's an example of how this can happen. If you tend to suffer increased flatulence whenever you get glutened, you might assume that increased flatulence on a particular day means that something you just ate contained gluten. You might then decide never to eat that particular food item again — forgetting that you ate baked beans earlier in the day. In this case, you might unnecessarily eliminate a nutritious item from your diet when you are simply suffering from the effect famously depicted in the film Blazing Saddles.

Another risk is that you interpret a normal variation in digestion as a sign of a food allergy or intolerance. But self-diagnosis is bad practice. Again, you risk unnecessarily eliminating nutritious items from your diet. If you suspect that you have a food allergy, ask your doctor to test for it. If you suspect lactose intolerance, read the next section.

Having said that, if you find that a given food consistently makes you feel unwell, avoid it even if the doctors can't find any reason for your reaction. Just don't jump to conclusions based on one bad experience and don't go looking for problems.

Your lactose intolerance might disappear

If you're celiac and lactose-intolerant, be aware that some celiacs are only temporarily lactose-intolerant. How can that be? Lactose, which is a sugar in milk, is digested in the small intestine by an enzyme called lactase. Lactase is not produced if the small intestine is damaged. The small intestine is damaged by celiac disease. A gluten-free diet allows the small intestine to heal. When it heals sufficiently to produce lactase, you can digest milk again. However, the healing process typically takes a few months.

If you have been avoiding dairy products due to temporary lactose intolerance and decide to try reintroducing them to your diet, wait until you have been on the gluten-free diet for four months. Start with small amounts of yogurt (which has less lactose than milk because some of it is pre-digested during fermentation), progressing gradually to larger amounts and then to cream and soft cheese and finally to hard cheese and milk.

Some people are permanently lactose intolerant. If you suspect this applies to you, ask your doctor for a test. Don't permanently give up dairy products on a whim. Celiacs need more, not less, calcium than "normal" people.

They sort of know whether you are sticking to the diet

If you have celiac disease, the markers of the disease in your blood should decrease as the diet takes effect. This means that your doctor can sort of tell whether you're sticking to the diet by ordering a blood test — only "sort of" because none of the various biomarkers used to test for celiac disease is perfectly correlated with gluten exposure. If you believe that you are following the diet but your blood tests do not show improvement or you continue to have symptoms, a dietitian can examine your diet in detail to help you identify the source of any remaining gluten.

Chapter 2: Identifying and avoiding gluten

The necessary first step when going gluten-free is learning to identify what foods contain gluten and where gluten might be hiding.

Gluten identification is a bit like bird identification. You become confident that you can recognize a particular bird. But then you find out that its plumage is different in summer than in winter, that the males and females are different colours, that it looks totally different when in flight, that it occupies the same habitat as a similar but different bird, and that its song is almost indistinguishable from that of an unrelated bird.

Similarly, a wheat-based carrot cake and a gluten-free carrot cake have the same colouring and hang out in the same places and even sound the same. (You know how you can sometimes hear them call out "buy me"?) Couscous looks like quinoa and not like other forms of wheat, but it's wheat. Buckwheat sounds like wheat, but it's not. If a restaurant offers a choice of regular bread or gluten-free bread with the soup, you can generally verify that they've served you the gluten-free bread because it falls apart easily and doesn't fly, but some restaurants manage to make gluten-free bread that hangs together fairly well.

Incidentally, the wheatear bird has nothing to do with wheat. According to Collins English Dictionary, *wheatear* probably comes from WHITE+ARSE; compare Dutch *witstaart*, French *culblanc*, white tail. This bird is actually white at the rear end, not on the ears. As with bird identification, so with gluten identification: it's easier if you are able to tell your arse from your elbow.

The gluten roll: food and drink list

This section contains a list of foods and drinks, each categorised as "YES", "NO", or "MAYBE".

- "YES" means that the food is naturally gluten-free and thus allowed on a gluten-free diet.

- "NO" means that the food has gluten-containing ingredients and thus not allowed on a gluten-free diet.

- "MAYBE" means that the food may or may not contain gluten, depending on the recipe and the manufacturing process. Check the label or, in a restaurant or other food business, check the menu or ask the server.

Inclusion in the "YES" category says nothing about whether the food is part of a healthy diet. For example, monosodium glutamate is marked as "YES" because you may see it on a label or you may suspect that it's in a meal in a restaurant and you need to know whether it's OK from the perspective of being gluten-free. But I am certainly not suggesting that you seek out foods containing monosodium glutamate.

If a food is gluten-free when it's fresh, it's usually also gluten-free if it has been frozen, dried, smoked, pickled, canned, bottled, packeted, or juiced — provided no other ingredients have been added in the process. For example, frozen peas, smoked haddock, and packets of nuts are fine. Canned fish, however, has to be soaked in something within the can. If that something is water, brine, or oil, it's still gluten-free. If that something is a sauce, you have to check the label. And a pre-packed fish pie is obviously a totally different kettle of fish.

Inclusion in the "NO" category applies to the *normal* versions of the relevant foods, for example, normal wheat bread or rye bread and normal barley-based beer. However, you may have special gluten-free versions of such products. For example, you may have bread made from gluten-free flours and starches. And you may have gluten-free beers, which are made from either a non-gluten grain or barley from which the gluten has been removed.

Inclusion in the "MAYBE" category applies to the *normal* versions of foods bought in shops, restaurants, and takeaways rather than special gluten-free versions or homemade food. For example, a homemade burger made with minced beef, onions, and herbs is fine. But some commercially produced burgers are padded out with wheat.

In general, the list contains categories like "fruits", "meats", and "nuts" rather than individual fruits, meats, and nuts. However, individual cereals and pseudo-cereals are listed because newcomers to the gluten-free diet are sometimes uncertain as to whether they are allowed. Also, a lot of misinformation about these foods is in circulation.

Ale. NO.

Amaranth. YES.

Arrowroot. YES.

Artificial sweeteners. MAYBE.

Baking powder. NO.

Barley. NO.

Battered food. NO. So no banana fritters, battered fish, onion rings in batter, or toad-in-the-hole.

Beansprouts. MAYBE. Some packets of fresh beansprouts say not suitable for people with wheat allergies.

Beer. NO. That includes ale, lager, and stout.

Berries. YES.

Bicarbonate of soda (baking soda). YES.

Biscuits. NO.

Bread. NO. Not in any form (loaves, rolls, flatbreads, wraps, etc.) or any colour (white, brown, black).

Breadcrumbed food. NO. So no breaded ham, rissoles, fishcakes, scampi in breadcrumbs, Scotch eggs.

Breakfast cereals. NO. Among normal products, even rice cereals usually contain barley and/or wheat.

Bubble tea. YES. The pearls are tapioca pearls.

Buckwheat. YES.

Burgers. MAYBE. Without a bun (which is not necessary anyway because burgers are typically served with other carbohydrates such as chips).

Butter. YES. Including buttermilk and ghee.

Cakes. NO.

Cheese, natural. YES.

Cheese, processed. MAYBE. Mostly OK in Europe. In America, you can get cheese in a spray can. Even such weird forms of cheese are usually gluten-free, but check.

Cheesecake. NO.

Chestnut. YES. Including chestnut flour.

Chewing gum. MAYBE. You could absorb any gluten in it, even though you don't swallow it.

Chickpea flour (gram flour). YES.

Chips (French fries). MAYBE. Many frozen chips are invisibly coated in wheat flour, and restaurants often cook fresh chips in the same oil as battered fish or breadcrumbed food.

Chocolate. MAYBE.

Chutney. MAYBE.

Cider. YES.

Codex wheat starch. YES. But not regular wheat starch.

Coffee. YES.

Confectionery. MAYBE.

Cooking fats. YES. But check the label if buying packet suet.

Cordials. YES.

Cornflour (cornstarch). YES.

Couscous. NO.

Crackers. NO.

Cream of tartar. YES.

Cream, natural. YES.

Cream, synthetic. MAYBE.

Crispbreads. NO.

Crisps. MAYBE.

Croissants. NO.

Crumbles. NO.

Custard. MAYBE.

Desserts. MAYBE.

Dextrin, dextrose, maltodextrin. YES. Does not contain barley malt. Even if derived from wheat, no gluten remains.

Dumplings. NO.

Eggs. YES.

Fish. YES.

Flavourings. YES. Very rarely contain gluten. If they do, the label should say so.

Flowers, edible. YES.

Food colouring. YES.

Fruits. YES.

Game birds. YES.

Ginger beer. YES.

Glucose syrup. YES.

Glutinous rice (a.k.a. sticky rice). YES. Misleading name; does not contain gluten. A type of white short-grain rice, so called because it becomes gluey when cooked (due to its high level of amylopectin).

Golden syrup. YES.

Gravy. MAYBE.

Gums and gelling agents. YES. Including guar gum, carrageenan, gelatin, xanthan gum.

Haggis. NO. Contains oats, which are usually contaminated with gluten from other grains.

Herbal teas (tisanes). YES.

Herbs. YES.

Honey. YES.

Hot chocolate. MAYBE.

Hotpot. MAYBE. May contain pearl barley.

Hummus. MAYBE.

Hydrolyzed wheat protein. NO.

Ice cream. MAYBE.

Jam. YES.

Jelly. YES.

Kvass. NO. Contains rye.

Legumes. YES.

Liqueurs (liquors). YES.

Macaroons. YES.

Maize. YES.

Malt. NO. Usually made from barley. So no malt extract, malt syrup, or malt flavouring.

Maple syrup. YES. Assuming that it is actually maple syrup and not maple-flavoured syrup.

Margarine. YES.

Marmalade. YES.

Marzipan. MAYBE.

Mayonnaise. MAYBE.

Meat. YES.

Meringue. YES.

Milk. YES. Including milkshakes, smoothies.

Millet. YES.

Miso. MAYBE. Some miso pastes are made from barley.

Mock meats. NO. Usually no, but check the label if you want this stuff.

Molasses (a.k.a. treacle). YES.

Monosodium glutamate. YES.

Mouldy Old Dough (Lieutenant Pigeon). YES. Very good novelty song.

Mustard condiments. MAYBE.

Mustard seeds. YES.

Noodles. MAYBE. Most noodles are made from wheat, but most rice noodles are gluten-free.

Nuts. YES. Including nut butters and ground almonds.

Oats. MAYBE. Only if they have the "gluten-free" label (most oats being contaminated with wheat gluten). Applies to all products containing oats, including oat milk and oat-based snack foods.

Oils. YES.

Pancakes. NO.

Pasta. NO. Most pasta is made from wheat, though pasta made from rice, buckwheat, etc., is usually gluten-free.

Pastry. NO.

Pate. MAYBE.

Pepper (a.k.a. bell pepper, sweet pepper, capsicum). YES.

Pickles. MAYBE.

Pies and pie-like things. NO. So no pasties, tarts, flans, quiches, sausage rolls, vol-au-vents.

Pizza. NO.

Polenta. YES.

Popcorn. MAYBE. But please be considerate and don't spoil other people's enjoyment of films with it.

Porridge. NO.

Potato. YES. Including potato starch, potato flour. But see also Chips.

Poultry. YES.

Pretzels. NO.

Puddings. MAYBE.

Quinoa. YES.

Quorn. MAYBE.

Ready meals. MAYBE.

Rice. YES. Including plain rice cakes, rice flour, ground rice, rice wine. But some sushi rice contains vinegar with gluten.

Rice milk. MAYBE.

Risotto. MAYBE. Depends on whether the stock is gluten-free.

Rusk. NO.

Rye. NO.

Sago. YES.

Salad vegetables. YES.

Samosas. NO.

Sauce mixes. MAYBE.

Sauces. MAYBE. Depends on whether any stock, soy sauce, or thickener in it has gluten.

Sausages. MAYBE.

Scones. NO.

Seasonings. MAYBE.

Seaweed and sea vegetables. YES.

Seeds. YES. Including seed-based confections such as halva and seed butters such as tahini.

Seitan. NO.

Semolina. NO.

Shellfish. YES.

Soft drinks and sodas. YES.

Sorbet. YES.

Sorghum. YES.

Soup. MAYBE. May contain pearl barley, wheat flour, wheat noodles, wheat croutons.

Soybean. YES. Including soy flour, soy lecithin, and tofu.

Soymilk. MAYBE.

Soy sauce. MAYBE. All soy sauces except tamari contain wheat.

Spices. YES.

Spirits. YES. Some celiacs report that some or all whisky drinks (a.k.a. whiskey or Scotch or bourbon) disagree with them, though manufacturers usually claim that distillation removes the gluten from the barley or rye.

Spreads. MAYBE.

Spring rolls. MAYBE. OK if the wrapper is made with rice flour, not if made with wheat.

Squash (drink). YES. Except barley squash.

Squash (food, a.k.a. pumpkin, gourd). YES.

Stew. MAYBE. May contain pearl barley.

Stock cubes and liquids. MAYBE.

Stuffing. MAYBE.

Sugar. YES.

Sushi. MAYBE.

Tabbouleh. NO. Contains bulgur wheat.

Tapioca (a.k.a. cassava, manioc). YES.

Taramasalata. MAYBE.

Tea. YES.

Teff. YES.

Tempura. NO.

Textured vegetable protein. MAYBE.

Tisanes. YES.

Vanilla. YES.

Vegetables. YES.

Vine leaves. YES. Including stuffed vine leaves or dolma, provided the stuffing is gluten-free.

Vinegar. MAYBE.

Wafers. NO.

Waffles. NO.

Welsh Rarebit. NO. Contains ale or other beer.

Wheat. NO.

Wheat berry. NO.

Wheatgrass. MAYBE. The young grass of the wheat plant, before it matures and yields grain. Doesn't contain gluten. But juiced or powdered wheatgrass products sometimes contain added wheat grain.

Wild rice. YES.

Wine. YES. Including fortified wines such as sherry and port.

Yeast. MAYBE. Baker's yeast is nearly always gluten-free, though check the label. Brewer's yeast is a by-product of beer brewing, contaminated with barley.

Yogurt. YES. Including natural and fruit yogurts (but obviously excluding those with granola toppings).

Yorkshire pudding. NO.

Zabaglione. YES. Without biscuits.

A gluten dose by any other name

What's in a name? That which we call barley, rye, or wheat by any other name would swell you as you eat.

It's useful to be aware of the other names, in case you're buying food in a country where non-wheat gluten doesn't have to be declared on the label or you're buying loose food.

Wheat (scientific name *Triticum*). The following are all varieties of, or parts of, the wheat plant: bulgur wheat, couscous, durum wheat, einkorn, emmer, farina, fasso, freekeh, graham flour, Kamut (from Khorasan wheat), mograbieh, seitan, semolina, spelt (also known as dinkel wheat). Note that seitan is basically wheat from which everything has been removed *except* the gluten; it's a big glob of gluten. This is the worst thing you could eat. It is the main ingredient in mock duck and in some other mock meats in some Asian and vegetarian cuisines (but not in Mock Turtle).

Barley (scientific name *Hordeum vulgare*). In the UK, most food and drink products containing barley helpfully have "barley" not only in the ingredients list but also in the name, for example, Barley Water, Barley Wine, Barleycup, Barley Flakes, Barley Malt Extract, Pearl Barley, Oat and Barley Porridge. Also look out for barley malt as an ingredient of other products.

Rye (scientific name *Secale cereale*). Food and drink containing rye is also easy to spot because rye has no other names (at least, not in English) and it will be in the ingredients list.

Hybrids. Triticale is a hybrid of wheat and rye.

Groats. These are hulled and crushed grains. If the grain is wheat, rye, barley, or oats not labelled as "gluten-free", you can't have it. If the grain is a gluten-free one such as buckwheat, you can have it (unless the label warns of possible contamination).

A gluten dose by contamination

You have to check the label on cereals such as oats and pseudo-cereals such as buckwheat, even though they do not naturally contain gluten. You have to be aware of what can happen in restaurant kitchens during the preparation of gluten-free meals. You even have to be attentive to what's happening in your own kitchen. Otherwise, you might inadvertently eat food that started out as gluten-free but has become contaminated with gluten. Given that even a small amount of gluten can be harmful to people with celiac disease or wheat allergy, avoiding contamination is important.

Cross-contamination is a minefield. Actually, it's more likely a cultivated field in which a gluten-free grain is grown close to wheat or in rotation with wheat; contamination can occur during growing and harvesting. Milling provides another opportunity for gluten contamination, if different grains are milled on the same equipment. Contamination of food products is also possible during weighing, packing, storage, manufacturing, and transportation, unless care is taken to avoid this.

Let's suppose that a foodstuff gets from a field to a grocery store without contamination. To prevent contamination at this point, the store should stack the gluten-free flour on a separate shelf from the wheat flour and should stack the gluten-free bread on a separate shelf from the wheat bread. The reason is that it's not uncommon for bags to split open or to have holes in them. Furthermore, some particularly sensitive celiacs say they get reactions if they eat gluten-free food that has been stacked next to gluten-containing food.

Now let's suppose that a foodstuff gets from a field or a sea to a restaurant kitchen without contamination. To prevent contamination at this point, restaurants will ideally have a separate kitchen for making gluten-free dishes or have separate timeslots for gluten-free dishes, with a thorough cleaning before the gluten-free slot. If kitchen staff must use the same kitchen at the same time for preparing all dishes, they must take extra care. For example, they must use separate chopping boards and knives and they must not fry the ingredients for a gluten-free dish in oil that has been used for frying gluten-containing foods. Good restaurants and delicatessens are aware of these and other measures that must be taken to ensure a dish is gluten-free. If you have any doubts, do ask for assurance that appropriate measures are being taken in the kitchen to avoid contamination.

Now let's suppose that a bottled sauce or some butter gets from a restaurant kitchen to your table without contamination. If the sauce bottle has a wide opening, be aware that a previous customer might have loosened some recalcitrant sauce from it using a knife already used for cutting wheat toast. If the butter is in an open dish, be aware that another customer might have double-dipped — used a knife to butter a wheat roll and then dipped the same knife back into the dish for more. This is actually very common, and the other customer might be at your own table. It could be someone who appears well-mannered in other respects. If gluten contamination of an accompaniment is a possibility and you really want it, ask whether it is available in an individual packet or ask for a fresh supply. (Something else to consider from a hygiene perspective: if an accompaniment may be contaminated with gluten, what else might it be contaminated with?)

Finally, let's suppose that a foodstuff gets as far as your own home without contamination. If you live with anyone who isn't on the gluten-free diet, cross-contamination can occur at home. Here are ways to avoid it.

- When chopping boards and utensils have been used to prepare gluten-containing food, wash them before using them for gluten-free food preparation.

- If you handle gluten-containing comestibles while preparing meals for others, wash your hands immediately afterward. This avoids transferring the gluten to your own food or to your mouth.

- Avoid making dishes for others using wheat, rye, or barley flour because this inevitably involves getting clouds of flour in the air and dough on your fingers, making accidental ingestion a distinct possibility. If you must make such dishes for others, consider wearing a mouth-guarding face mask.

- Consider having separate cupboards, or at least separate shelves within a cupboard, for gluten-containing and gluten-free foods.

- Ensure that the "normal" people in the household know that, whenever they use a knife to spread butter or something from a jar onto their bread or crackers, they must not dip the same knife back into the food container.

- Don't share a soup, dip, or fondue with people who are dipping wheat bread into it.

- Don't share a toaster with your normal housemates because their breadcrumbs are inevitably left in the toaster and are sure to contaminate your gluten-free bread. If you use a toaster, have a separate one. Alternatively, use the grill. On a grill, you can toast both normal and gluten-free bread at the same time by placing them well away from each other on the wire rack. Also, it's easier to wash the rack in between uses than to keep a toaster clean, and the grill doesn't take up extra space on the worktop.

Although the risk of contamination must be taken seriously, it must be assessed in context. Here are two examples.

In a cafe, I asked whether the macaroons were gluten-free. (Macaroons should, of course, be made with ground almonds rather than flour, making them excellent little gluten-free sweet treats, but one has to ask in case a nonstandard recipe has been used.). I was told that they have no gluten-containing ingredients but are made in the same kitchen as the other baked goods. I judged the risk of contamination to be low and happily ate a macaroon.

In a restaurant, I asked whether the chips were gluten-free. I was told that they have no gluten-containing ingredients but are fried in the same oil as the fishcakes, which are coated in breadcrumbs. I judged that contamination was certain; the oil will contain great globs of gluten, and the chips will then be thoroughly coated in that oil. I forewent the chips.

A gluten dose put to the test

There are gluten detectors, apart from the one in your body. Kits are available for home use. Although they are too expensive for routine use, it could be worth getting a 2-test or 5-test kit, for use in a couple of situations. First, if there's a particular food product that you plan to eat frequently and you are unsure whether it contains gluten, you could test one sample (though you couldn't be sure that other batches of the same product are the exactly the same). Second, if you believe you have been glutened by food sold as gluten-free, you could test it. If it's restaurant food, you would have to take some home with you in a doggie bag.

The official language of gluten

What do you like to read? Science fiction? Biography? Philosophy? Economics? Short stories? Comic books? Historical romances? Obituaries? Food labels, anyone?

The first few food shopping trips when you go gluten-free take much longer than usual because you have to read the labels on everything you would like to buy. And you might find it frustrating because you will have to put one item after another back on the shelf, due to the gluten content. Within a few weeks, however, you will be able to shop quickly again because (1) you will be expert at reading labels, and (2) you will have identified certain brands of certain products that you can have.

Gluten-free labelling for special dietary foods

Many countries base their regulations about gluten composition and labelling on the **international Codex standard** for foods for special dietary use for persons intolerant to gluten. The main provisions of this standard are as follows.[1]

- Foods may be labelled as "gluten-free" if the gluten level does not exceed 20 mg/kg (that is, 20 parts per million). This applies to products that are specially formulated for people intolerant to gluten *and* made from *either* non-gluten-containing ingredients *or* ingredients from wheat, rye, or barley that have been processed to reduce the gluten to the required level. This means that it applies not only to bread containing a gluten-free flour mix instead of wheat flour but also to bread containing wheat flour in which the gluten has been reduced to less than 20 ppm. The latter is typically listed in the ingredients as "Codex wheat starch". This is safe for most celiacs but may not be suitable for those who are allergic to something in wheat besides gluten.

- For foods with gluten-containing ingredients that have been processed to reduce the gluten content to a level above 20 ppm up to 100 ppm, the labelling is determined at national level.

- The labelling of uncontaminated oats is determined at national level.

Let's look at how the Codex standard has been used in shaping the European and American regulations.

The EU regulation about gluten-free foods is based on the Codex standard, adopting the 20 ppm and 100 ppm levels. The main provisions of this regulation are as follows.[2]

- The statement "gluten-free" may be made only for food containing no more than 20 ppm of gluten.

- The statement "very low gluten" may be made only for food which has gluten-containing ingredients but which has been specially processed to reduce the gluten to no more than 100 ppm.

- These statements may be accompanied by the statements "suitable for people intolerant to gluten" or "suitable for coeliacs".

- These statements may be accompanied by the statements "specifically formulated for people intolerant to gluten" or "specifically formulated for coeliacs" if the food has been specially produced, prepared, or processed to reduce the gluten content of gluten-containing ingredients or to substitute gluten-containing ingredients with other ingredients naturally free of gluten.

- Oats in food presented as gluten-free or very low gluten must be produced in a way to avoid gluten contamination, and the gluten content of such oats must not exceed 20 ppm.

- The regulation applies to all foodstuffs, including non-pre-packed food.

The US Food and Drug Administration (FDA) rule defining the use of the term "gluten-free" on food labels uses only the 20 ppm level. The main provisions of this rule are as follows.[3]

- The term "gluten-free" may be used for any food that is inherently gluten-free or does not contain any gluten-containing grain or is derived from a gluten-containing grain that has been processed to remove the gluten to the required level. Any unavoidable presence of gluten in the food must be less than 20 ppm.

- Foods that meet the definition of "gluten-free" may be labelled as "gluten-free" but are not required to be so labelled.

- Oats marketed as "gluten-free" must contain less than 20 ppm of gluten.

- The rule applies to FDA-regulated packaged foods and dietary supplements. It does *not* apply to foods regulated by the U.S. Department of Agriculture (USDA) or the Alcohol and Tobacco Tax Trade Bureau (TTB) — that is, it does not apply to meat, poultry, eggs, and alcohol.

There's an interesting omission from both the EU and the US regulations compared to the Codex standard: if a gluten-free product is a substitute for an important basic food, it should supply approximately the same amount of vitamins and minerals as the food it replaces. Even in the Codex standard, there's nothing to say that a gluten-free product can't be loaded with salt, sugar, artificial sweeteners, artificial colours, and so on. So don't get to thinking that "gluten-free" equates to "healthy".

Allergen labelling for normal foods

For normal foods, there are many national differences regarding food labelling in general and the identification of allergens in particular. This section summarizes the rules on allergen labelling in the EU and the US.

The EU regulation on the provision of food information to consumers (sometimes abbreviated to FIC) covers allergen labelling as well as other information, including nutrition declarations.[4]

The regulation applies to the following 14 allergens: cereals containing gluten, crustaceans, eggs, fish, peanuts, soybeans, milk, nuts, celery, mustard, sesame, sulphites, lupin, and molluscs. We're interested in the first one — cereals containing gluten. The main provisions of the regulation regarding all 14 allergens are as follows.

- For pre-packed foods, the list of ingredients must emphasize the presence of any of the 14 allergens. Most food producers have chosen to use bold type for this purpose but they could use italics, underlining, or a different background colour. If an ingredient is a variety or form of wheat that doesn't have "wheat" in its name, the producer must indicate that it comes from wheat. For example, couscous in a pre-packed salad is listed as "couscous (from **wheat**)". It's the same for other allergens, for example, "whey (**milk**)". If there is no list of ingredients (if the packaging is too small or if certain other exceptions apply), the presence of an allergen must be indicated by the word "contains" followed by the name of the allergen. In the UK, the FSA is extending the FIC labelling requirement to foods packed on site for direct sale to consumers (for example, in a deli), effective October 2021.

- For non-prepacked food, e.g. food packed at a consumer's request or provided as a free sample or complimentary snack, allergen information must be available. Member states can make their own rules regarding the form of this information. In the UK, allergen information (but not a full ingredients list) must be available in an accessible manner, such as by asking a member of staff.

- For foods offered for sale by distance selling, information on the allergens must be available before the purchase is concluded.

- Information must be in a language easily understood by the consumers of the member states where a food is marketed.

The aim of the Food Information for Consumers regulation is to make allergen labelling simpler by putting all the allergen information in one place, namely, the list of ingredients. But it seems to be a retrograde step in some respects.

First, producers may only name the ingredients, not the allergenic protein within an ingredient. The old "contains gluten" statement has gone. It is now incumbent on you to know which ingredients contain gluten (wheat, rye, and barley).

Second, the *definite* presence of an allergen can be indicated *only* by emphasis in the ingredients list. The allergy boxes that some manufacturers previously put after the ingredients lists are replaced with a statement like "For allergens, see ingredients in bold". Therefore, you must look at the list of ingredients.

Third, information about the possibility of the *unintentional* presence of gluten (or other allergens) is not adequately regulated. Producers can voluntarily provide a "may contain gluten" statement or other advisory statement, but there are no rules on when an advisory statement should be provided or what form it should take.

Now let's look at some real labels, starting with one for a fish pie:

"Potato, fresh semi-skimmed **milk**, cod (14%) (**fish**), salmon (9%) (**fish**), fresh whipping cream (**milk**), butter (**milk**), smoked haddock (3%) (**fish**), **wheat** flour, fresh single cream (**milk**), spinach, Cheddar cheese (**milk**), breadcrumbs (**wheat** flour, yeast, salt, colours (plain caramel, paprika extract), turmeric extract, sunflower oil), free range **egg** yolk, fresh parsley, salt, **fish** stock (cod (**fish**), anchovy paste (**fish**), potato flakes, salt, lemon juice, onion powder, sunflower oil), lemon juice, white pepper.

Allergy information

For allergens, including cereals containing gluten, see ingredients in bold. May also contain nuts, peanuts and sesame. Although we do our very best to take out all the bones, some may remain."

How easy was it for you to spot the gluten in the ingredients list? There are two gluten-containing ingredients. If you found it difficult, it's because overuse of emphasis actually dilutes the message. This is a problem for products containing many allergenic ingredients — especially for fish pies, where every fish has to be marked as such. I can sort of understand the reasoning; everyone knows that salmon is fish, but I guess that some people do not know whether "hake" is a fish, a crustacean, a cereal, a nut, or a form of Japanese poetry.

This label is on a packet of fruit & nut mix:

"Ingredients: **PEANUTS**, Raisins (Raisins, Vegetable Oil), Sultanas, **BRAZIL NUTS, ALMONDS, CASHEWS**.

Allergy Advice: For Allergens Including Cereals Containing Gluten, See Ingredients in BOLD. Also, May Contain Other Nuts and Sesame."

Your eye is caught by the phrase "Allergy Advice", which tells you to see the ingredients list. So you go to the ingredients list and look out for cereals containing gluten in bold — but there are no gluten-containing cereals in the list. It's just a standard statement, wasting your time. (Furthermore, the bold face in the font used on this particular label is barely bolder than the regular face, so the most noticeable thing about the allergen names is that they are in uppercase. Thus, the instruction to see the ingredients in BOLD serves as a variant of the Stroop test.)

The good thing about the regulation is that it applies to all food products and to all types of food retailers and caterers and to all methods of selling, whereas the previous regulation did not apply to loose foods.

Another good thing about the regulation is that it may cause some restaurants to re-think their menus. In response to the need to provide consistent information about allergens, many restaurants have produced an allergen card. This typically contains a table with the menu items listed in the left column and the allergens in the top row. The server fetches a copy of this when a customer asks about an allergen. One restaurant I visited had an extensive menu with dozens of items, covering breakfast, lunches, dinners, and snacks. But a scan of the relevant column on the allergen card revealed only two gluten-free dishes, one of which would be too spicy for me. So it was lamb or nothing for me. I like lamb, but I would have appreciated a choice of dishes and won't go there again. Perhaps the process of compiling such a table will make some restaurant proprietors realize that people of the gluten-free persuasion are unlikely to dine there.

The US legislation on allergen information is the *Food Allergen Labeling and Consumer Protection Act*, sometimes abbreviated to FALCPA.[5]

FALCPA applies to the following eight allergens: milk, eggs, fish, Crustacean shellfish, tree nuts, wheat, peanuts, soybeans. The main provisions regarding all eight allergens are as follows.

- On labels for packaged food, the presence of one of the allergens or a protein derived from one of the allergens must be indicated in one of two ways: (1) In a "Contains" statement after the list of ingredients, for example, "Contains wheat", or (2) In parentheses after the name of the food from which the allergen is derived, for example, "flour (wheat)".

- The font size used for the allergen information must be no smaller than the size used in the ingredients list. (There is no requirement for allergen information to be in bold type, though some manufacturers do emphasize the text in bold or in other ways.)

Although FALCPA is helpful in some respects, it falls short of consumer expectations in other respects.

First, and most importantly for our purposes, there is no requirement to declare gluten from sources other than wheat; gluten derived from rye, barley, or impure oats does not have to be declared. Check whether the ingredients list includes rye or barley. If still unsure, ask the manufacturer or find a brand of the same foodstuff explicitly labelled as "gluten-free".

Second, you have to look at both the ingredients list and the "Contains" statement. The ingredients list could include "Couscous (precooked semolina)". If you're knowledgeable about the various guises of wheat (if you've read up to this point in this book and memorized it all ready for the test), you'll recognize both "couscous" and "semolina" as no-nos. But if you can't remember the names of all the possible guises of wheat when you're shopping, you have to rely on the "Contains wheat" statement.

Third, it does not apply to loose foods — sandwiches placed in a wrapper in response to a person's order, food sold by street vendors or at festivals, and so on.

Finally, food producers are not required to provide statements about the possibility of the unintentional presence of gluten (or other allergens), though they can voluntarily provide a "may contain" statement or other advisory statement.

Advisory labelling

As mentioned in the previous section, information about the unintentional presence of gluten from contact with other foods is not adequately regulated in either the EU or the US. Food producers can voluntarily provide an advisory statement ("may contain...", for example) but there are no rules on when such a statement should be provided or what form it should take.

The regulators know that this is an issue. The EU regulation enables the European Commission to implement further rules on this, and the US regulation says that someone should investigate it and submit a report. However, as at early 2020, there is no news on either side of the pond about any definite plans for rules on advisory statements.

What do the voluntary advisory labels mean in practice? In 2012–2013, a UK study analyzed allergen labelling and allergen content of samples of food products in which the allergens were *not* intentional ingredients. The percentage of samples with detectable gluten was 6.1%.[6] The percentage of samples with detectable gluten but no advisory label was 3.3%. The percentage of samples with no detectable gluten and an advisory label was 19%. There was no correlation between the level of allergen detected and the severity of the wording on the label.

Similar studies in the US found that advisory labels for wheat or gluten on products not labelled gluten-free but appearing to be free of gluten-containing ingredients were not a useful predictor of gluten content.[7]

The situation becomes even less clear when product information is inconsistent. A particular chocolate bar has a "may also contain wheat" statement, on both the wrapper and the manufacturer's website. The website also contains recipes. One of the recipes is for "gluten free cookies". The recipe calls for a quantity of chocolate and parenthetically adds that their own chocolate bar is their favourite for this purpose, linking to the page that includes the "may contain" statement. I don't even know whether this conforms to regulations. It would definitely be wrong to put a "gluten-free" claim on the product label, but is it wrong to reference it in a recipe with "gluten-free" in the name? If the recipe were on someone else's website, it would presumably be OK because the manufacturer could not be held liable for other people's express or implied statements about their products. Is it significant from a regulatory perspective that the recipe is on the manufacturer's own website?

In view of this unsatisfactory situation, I have two recommendations: (1) Don't read anything into the exact phrasing of advisory statements ("may contain...", "may contain traces of...", "produced in a factory that handles...", and so on), and (2) To spread the risk of gluten contamination, limit your intake of "may contain" foods and don't eat the same "may contain" food frequently. If you're very sensitive to gluten, it's best to avoid "may contain" foods altogether, even though they often don't contain gluten.

Gluten-free vs. wheat-free vs. Free From

Food labelled as "gluten-free" is not necessarily free from wheat; it may contain wheat starch that has been processed to reduce the gluten to less than 20 parts per million. This is typically listed in the ingredients as "Codex wheat starch" because it complies with the Codex standard for gluten-free labelling.

Conversely, food described as "wheat-free" is not necessarily free from gluten; rye and barley also contain gluten.

In the UK, many food shops have "Free From" shelves, but the food on these shelves is not necessarily free from either gluten or wheat. It may be there because it's free from nuts, milk, or other allergens. Rye bread can be there because it's wheat-free though not gluten-free. And normal food might have been stacked in the Free From section by mistake. (I have seen this — and reported it to the store manager, for which I was thanked.) Furthermore, the term "Free From" has no legal definition. *Even in the Free From section, you have to read the labels.*

Although the "Free From" section of a supermarket or its website contains a selection of products that are free from particular ingredients, most other sections of the store contain naturally gluten-free food too. Furthermore, the other sections may have processed food products that don't contain gluten even though not explicitly marketed as "gluten-free", and these products are sometimes cheaper than their counterparts in the "Free From" section. The cynical part of me thinks that "Free From" is something that supermarkets write on a sign as another way of saying "feak and weeble people and food faddists this way", just as they have signs at the checkouts for basket cases.

Labelling for medicinal products

Most medicines contain either no gluten or virtually no gluten (less than the amount that could be found in food legitimately labelled as gluten-free). But getting information about gluten content is more difficult for medicines than for food because the labelling regulations for medicines generally do not cover gluten. However, the FDA has published draft guidance on gluten labelling for oral drug products.[8] According to this guidance, producers may voluntarily include a statement that their drug "contains no ingredient made from a gluten-containing grain (wheat, barley or rye)" when such a statement is truthful.

If you think you are getting glutened by a medicine, note that some side effects of some medicines are similar to some symptoms of gluten-related disorders; it's much more likely that what you are experiencing is a side effect than a gluten reaction.

The magical quantity 20 ppm plus 80

The tour of the official language of gluten will finish by considering why 20 parts per million is the upper level required for the "gluten-free" label.

This level is equivalent to 20 minutes in about two years. Imagine being in pain 20 times over a 2-year period, each time for only one minute. You will probably conclude that you would hardly notice the pain. So surely a bit more than 20 ppm of gluten in food would be of no consequence?

Well, the level in the previous version of the Codex standard was 200 ppm. It was reduced to 20 ppm after a multicentre trial coordinated from the University of Maryland School of Medicine established 20 ppm as the safe level; celiacs who had already been on the gluten-free diet for at least two years and who were "challenged" with 50 mg of gluten per day for three months suffered measurable damage to the intestinal villi.[9] This damage did not happen with celiacs challenged with 10 mg of gluten per day or with the placebo (no gluten) group. The conclusion was that 200 ppm is not safe because the harmful intake of 50 mg per day could be reached with a consumption of 250 g per day of nominally gluten-free products, an amount consumed by many celiacs. 100 ppm (the current "very low gluten" level) was also judged unsafe because consumption of wheat substitute products by celiacs is sometimes as high as 500 g per day.

500 g per day. Gosh. That's the weight of a large loaf of gluten-free bread. I can't imagine eating a whole loaf in one day or the same weight in other wheat substitute products. The thought of eating that amount of wheat substitute products in a day blows my mind before it gets a chance to blow up my gut. But I'm not Italian. I'll come back to that point soon.

The introduction of the 20 ppm level was controversial but has worked out well. One advantage of the 20 ppm level is that it leaves room for a margin of error for those celiacs who are particularly sensitive. Only one person dropped out of the gluten challenge study due to a clinical relapse and that person was only being challenged with 10 mg of gluten per day, whereas most people in that group did not even suffer silent intestinal damage. Conversely, the majority of people in the 50 mg group did suffer intestinal damage but not clinical relapse. This means that damage can occur silently, and the long-term health implications of that are not known.

Fortunately, the 20 ppm level has proved to be achievable. Before its introduction, some people had worried that manufacturers would find it difficult to manufacture and test products to this level and would stop making gluten-free products. This has not happened.

A study published in 2013 examined the risk for celiacs of intestinal damage from intake of seven gluten-free food groups (bread, pasta, pastry, biscuits, pizza, breakfast cereals, and breadcrumb-coated food) at the population level in Italy, Spain, Germany, and Norway.[10] The study took into account three factors: the range of consumption of gluten-free products, the range of gluten concentration in these products, and the distribution of gluten thresholds among celiacs. The researchers purchased gluten-free wheat substitute products in local shops and tested them for gluten in January 2010 (that is, after the 20 ppm EU regulation had been published but before it had come into force, when manufacturers were preparing for the change). They found that 99.5% of the samples had less than 20 ppm of gluten, with most (94%) having a gluten level below the limit of the sensitivity of the test method (<5 ppm). They calculated that the percentage of the celiac population at risk of intestinal damage due to the consumption of gluten-free products was 0.01 in Germany, 0.02 in Norway, 0.05 in Spain, and 0.15 in Italy. The higher risk in Italy was related mainly to the higher consumption of wheat substitute products, mostly pasta, rather than the gluten levels in the products available there. The researchers concluded that gluten-free products in Europe are very safe and that more attention should be paid to other potential sources of gluten intake, such as restaurant meals and voluntary transgressions.

Talking of voluntary transgressions: don't do it. If food containing more than 20 ppm can be harmful to celiacs, whether silently or noisily, then deliberately eating food that actually has wheat, rye, or barley as an ingredient takes you into the realm of gluten for punishment.

You might think that ingredients that start out with no gluten (such as potato starch) would be safer than Codex wheat starch, which starts out with plenty of gluten. That is, you might think that the risk of failing to reduce the gluten in wheat starch would be greater than the risk of contaminating naturally gluten-free ingredients. But the European study found that most of the Codex wheat starch products were well within the limit for the "gluten-free" claim.

A glancing blow

Once you have identified gluten-free brands of the types of food products you buy regularly (whether naturally gluten-free or specially formulated to have the "gluten-free" label), don't get complacent. Food manufacturers can change their recipes at any time. Sometimes, a product that previously contained gluten becomes gluten-free. Conversely, a previously gluten-free product can degenerate into a no-go area. So, glance at the labels even for familiar products. You will soon be able to speed-read food labels, leaving you time to get back to reading your science fiction books or rock star biographies or whatever.

Chapter 3: Understanding gluten-free nutrition

Now you know how to identify gluten and thus how to eliminate it from your diet. But that's not enough. You deserve a diet that's not only free of gluten but also healthy. This chapter supplies the nutritional rationale for the dietary recommendations in the next chapter. If you want to start on the diet right now, skip to the next chapter. But it would be good to come back here sometime because this background information will help you to make healthy choices when planning meals.

Avoiding common mistakes

The worst thing since sliced bread

You can't simply give up a food group and not replace it with something else. Your first thought might be to toast a couple of slices of gluten-free bread for breakfast instead of toasting a couple of slices of wheat or rye bread. That would certainly replace the wheat or rye bread in terms of bulk. And the nutrition declarations on wheat loaves and gluten-free loaves are in many cases similar regarding the energy-providing nutrients — fats, carbohydrates, and protein — and consequently the total calories. So why not just replace one with the other?

One reason is that the ingredients of gluten-free bread have fewer vitamins and minerals. The main ingredients of wheat bread besides the yeast are wheat flour and some flour treatment agents. In gluten-free bread, the main ingredients are typically tapioca starch, potato starch or potato flour, and corn starch. It typically also contains xanthan gum, some additives, and a few baffling ingredients.

Tapioca starch comes from the root of the cassava plant. It has no A, B, C, D, or E vitamins, negligible minerals, very little protein, no fat, and negligible fibre. The starch provides a similar quantity of calories as wheat flour but cannot substitute for wheat flour in the diet due to the lack of nutrition. The problem is the opportunity cost. You will feel full from eating foods containing tapioca starch, such as gluten-free bread and cakes, but will not be adequately nourished. So you will either suffer malnutrition or you will eat something more nourishing in addition to the tapioca-based food, probably something that will come with its own payload of carbohydrates, and then you will get overweight or suffer energy swings. Furthermore, cassava contains cyanide. Most of this is removed during the processing that morphs it into tapioca starch, but it's a lot of processing to get something with empty calories at the end. Corn starch and potato starch also leave a lot to be desired in nutritional terms, though potato flour does have some nutrients, including B vitamins.

Some gluten-free people bemoan the fact that, in many countries, it is mandatory for wheat bread to be fortified with certain vitamins and minerals, whereas there is no such requirement for gluten-free bread. In the UK, for example, iron, thiamin (vitamin B1) and niacin (vitamin B3) must be added to all wheat bread, and calcium must be added to all non-wholemeal wheat bread.

Wheat fortification initiatives recognize the fact that many people get the majority of their carbohydrates — indeed, the majority of their total calories — from wheat. But that shouldn't be the case, not even for people who can tolerate gluten. For some people, breakfast is a couple of slices of toast, lunch is a thick baguette with only a thin layer of filling, a mid-afternoon snack is a couple of biscuits, and dinner is pasta or pizza with tomato sauce. If you subsisted like this before you were advised to go gluten-free, then your diet wasn't well balanced and it would be a bad idea to simply replace the wheat with gluten-free substitutes. A better idea is to reduce the amount of carbohydrates in your diet and choose foods that are more nourishing than gluten-free wheat substitutes, including vegetables, eggs, and dairy products. Then the lack of fortification in gluten-free bread will be of no concern to you.

Here's another reason to avoid simply replacing a wheat sandwich with a gluten-free sandwich. The sandwich was invented by John Montagu, the 4th Earl of Sandwich, in the 18th century to enable him to continue his game at the gambling table while eating his meal. Not needing to use any utensils, he had one hand free and clean for handling the playing cards. (Dishes combining bread with meat or other foods actually existed in England and elsewhere earlier, but sandwiching was popularised by the Earl.) In the 21st century, the practice of having a sandwich for lunch rather than a meal requiring a fork is used to tie office workers to their desks rather than the gambling table — often by the workers themselves rather than their employers. In the UK, anyone who works more than six hours a day is entitled to an uninterrupted 20-minute break. Contracts of employment may provide for a longer break. You should take the break you are entitled to because eating while working, or even eating while using your work computer for personal purposes, can be stressful and can interfere with digestion. Use the break to get away from your desk and eat a healthy meal. If your boss objects to this, point out that you are more productive after you have moved your body and cleared your mind.

Yet another reason to avoid simply replacing the wheat sandwich with a gluten-free sandwich relates to gut bacteria. There is a concern that a gluten-free diet can adversely affect the balance of good bacteria and bad bacteria. In a study in which ten healthy people went on a gluten-free diet for a month, good bacteria decreased and bad bacteria increased.[11] The author of this study acknowledges its limitations with respect to the small number of participants and the short duration. I have another concern, which is that the diet is reported as "replacing the gluten-containing foods they normally ate with certified gluten-free foods". This implies that wheat bread was simply replaced by processed gluten-free bread, and so on. As you know, this is not my idea of a healthy gluten-free diet. In fact, this is another reason for eating fewer processed gluten-free products and more vegetables. In the long-term, a diet with a high proportion of vegetables improves the diversity and abundance of good bacteria in the gut. Researchers in the field of gut bacteria have concluded that a balanced diet must include many more vegetables than the average American eats, given that less than half of Americans report eating vegetables at dinner and even fewer in lunch foods. [12]

You can have gluten-free bread occasionally. Sometimes, it's convenient. Some places, it's all that's on offer. Just don't make it a dietary staple.

When you do eat gluten-free bread, consider buying it from an artisan bakery or making it yourself in a bread machine. That way, you might get a more nutritious and less debased loaf. Which mainstream brand of gluten-free bread is best? When I went gluten-free, other celiacs told me that their preferred brand was better than the others. I would try a recommended brand and think "maybe it's better than such-and-such brand, but that's not saying much". I soon realized that my distaste for gluten-free bread was due to still having a memory of the taste and texture of wheat bread. This memory faded after a few weeks and then I simply compared the gluten-free breads with each other rather than with wheat bread. I concluded that most brands of gluten-free bread are similar in terms of palatability. So it's best to get whichever one currently has the healthiest list of ingredients and accept that even the best gluten-free bread will not closely resemble its wheaten counterpart because gluten is the quintessential component of bread.

White is the new brown

For bread, the "brown is healthiest" message is deeply ingrained, so to speak, in all of us. We all know that brown bread is made with flour that has been ground from the whole grain and thus contains more nutrients and fibre than white bread, which is made from refined flour. But this line of argument is irrelevant to gluten-free bread because the main ingredient is starch. If you compare the ingredients lists on the white and brown gluten-free loaves from the same manufacturer, you will find that the main ingredients are the same in both but some brown stuff has been added to the brown loaf to make it brown. And the brown stuff is usually something unhealthy, such as caramelised sugar.

Therefore, the white bread is actually healthier. Manufacturers of gluten-free bread offer brown bread because they know that some people have been conditioned to demand it. Resist. White is the new brown.

Replacing the work of wheat

A common concern with the gluten-free diet is where to get the nutrients provided by wheat. Another concern is what to slot into the diet at the places where wheat-based foods commonly sit. So we'll look at the work of wheat in terms of nutrition and uses. We'll see that quinoa, rice, and buckwheat together can do this work.

Note that if you ate more rye or barley than wheat before going gluten-free, this section is nonetheless applicable. Those cereals contain similar nutrients to wheat, though in varying proportions.

The nutritional work of wheat

After giving up wheat, where are we going to get its rich supply of B vitamins? This is a valid concern because B vitamins cannot be stored in the body and thus must be in the diet every day. Quinoa is your best friend for gluten-free B vitamins. Brown rice and buckwheat are also good friends. These three foods also provide most of the minerals in wheat and a similar amount of energy (calories).

For a finer-grained analysis of the situation with regard to vitamins and minerals, we'll look at nutritional comparisons of three wheat replacements — quinoa to replace couscous (in a main meal), brown rice flour to replace wheat flour (in baking), and buckwheat flour to replace wheat flour (in pancakes, for example).

The source of the data in the following comparison tables is the Canadian Nutrient File from Health Canada, which is largely based on the United States Department of Agriculture (USDA) nutrient database and is searchable at http://www.healthcanada.gc.ca/cnf. Vitamins and minerals are included in the tables if the quantity in either of the foods being compared is at least 5% of the recommended daily intake.

Quinoa (pronounced however you want to pronounce it) is a pseudo-cereal with a nutty taste. The following table compares the nutrition in cooked couscous and cooked quinoa. As you can see, quinoa compares favourably with couscous. It actually has more of most B vitamins and more iron and magnesium. The protein value is similar. Quinoa contains a good amount of essential amino acids and provides better quality protein than other gluten-free grains. Selenium is missing, but we'll get that covered elsewhere in the diet. In short, quinoa is a superb source of nutrients and fibre for people on a gluten-free diet. It's so good that the UN designated 2013 as the International Year of Quinoa, on the basis that it has a role in eradicating hunger, malnutrition, and poverty.

	Couscous, cooked, 100 g	Quinoa, cooked, 100 g
Calories	112	120
Fat	0 g	0 g
Carbohydrates	23 g	21 g
Protein	4 g	4 g
Fibre	1 g	3 g
Vitamin B1 (thiamin)	0.063 mg	0.107 mg
Vitamin B2 (riboflavin)	0.027 mg	0.110 mg
Vitamin B3 (niacin)	0.983 mg	0.412 mg
Vitamin B6 (pyridoxine)	0.051 mg	0.123 mg
Folate	15 mcg	42 mcg
Iron	0.38 mg	1.49 mg
Magnesium	8 mg	64 mg
Phosphorous	22 mg	152 mg
Potassium	58 mg	172 mg
Zinc	0.26 mg	1.09 mg
Copper	0.041 mg	0.192 mg
Manganese	0.084 mg	0.631 mg

	Couscous, cooked, 100 g	Quinoa, cooked, 100 g
Selenium	27.5 mcg	0

Brown rice flour compares fairly well with whole-grain wheat flour, as shown in the following table. The rice flour has more of some vitamins and minerals and less of others. However, there is less protein and less fibre and no selenium.

	Wheat flour, whole grain, 100 g	Rice flour, brown, 100 g
Calories	340	363
Fat	2 g	3 g
Carbohydrates	74 g	76 g
Protein	10 g	7 g
Fibre	13 g	5 g
Vitamin B1 (thiamin)	0.297 mg	0.443 mg
Vitamin B2 (riboflavin)	0.188 mg	0.080 mg
Vitamin B3 (niacin)	5.347 mg	6.340 mg
Vitamin B5 (pantothenic acid)	1.011 mg	1.591 mg
Vitamin B6 (pyridoxine)	0.191 mg	0.736 mg
Folate	28 mcg	16 mcg
Iron	3.71 mg	1.98 mg
Magnesium	117 mg	112 mg
Phosphorous	323 mg	337 mg
Potassium	394 mg	289 mg
Zinc	2.96 mg	2.45 mg
Copper	0.475 mg	0.230 mg
Manganese	3.999 mg	4.013 mg
Selenium	12.7 mcg	0

Buckwheat is a pseudo-cereal unrelated to wheat. The following table shows that buckwheat flour is very similar to wheat flour in terms of B vitamins and richer in vitamin K and magnesium. Again, selenium is significantly lower.

	Wheat flour, whole grain, 100 g	Buckwheat flour, whole groat, 100 g
Calories	340	335
Fat	2 g	3 g
Carbohydrates	74 g	71 g
Protein	10 g	13 g
Fibre	13 g	7 g
Vitamin B1 (thiamin)	0.297 mg	0.417 mg
Vitamin B2 (riboflavin)	0.188 mg	0.190 mg
Vitamin B3 (niacin)	5.347 mg	6.150 mg
Vitamin B5 (pantothenic acid)	1.011 mg	0.440 mg
Vitamin B6 (pyridoxine)	0.191 mg	0.582 mg
Vitamin K	1.9 mcg	7.0 mcg
Folate	28 mcg	54 mcg
Iron	3.71 mg	4.06 mg
Magnesium	117 mg	251 mg
Phosphorous	323 mg	337 mg
Potassium	394 mg	577 mg
Zinc	2.96 mg	3.12 mg
Copper	0.475 mg	0.515 mg
Manganese	3.999 mg	2.030 mg
Selenium	12.7 mcg	5.7 mcg

We have seen that quinoa, rice, and buckwheat together replace the nutrients in wheat, except for selenium. According to other nutrition data sources, there may actually be a small amount of selenium in quinoa and brown rice flour. Nonetheless, the foods that do the nutritional work of wheat in the gluten-free diet have low levels of selenium, whereas some wheat-based foods provide a significant percentage of the recommended intake. Do we need to do anything special about this? Maybe, maybe not. Selenium is an antioxidant, which means that it mops up free radicals and thus protects against some diseases. It also helps thyroid function. It is undoubtedly important. But the lack of wheat in your diet may not be the main factor in your selenium status, for two reasons.

First, not all wheat eaters get as much selenium as suggested by the preceding tables. The data is derived from an American database, and American wheat has ten times more selenium than British wheat. (Other North American wheat is also high in selenium, and other northern European wheat is also low in it.) Selenium intake in the UK roughly halved between the 1980s and 2000, dropping to below the recommended intake. One factor in this drop is believed to be the declining usage in bread-making of wheat imported from North America during that period.[13]

Second, you may be getting a high proportion of your selenium intake from non-cereal sources. Some other gluten-free foods have more selenium than wheat, namely, fish and shellfish and red and white meat. And there is a moderate amount of selenium in some other foods, including eggs, mushrooms, cashew nuts, cabbage, baked beans, and oats. If you regularly eat fish and meat and a selection of other selenium-containing foods, it may be that you already have enough selenium in your diet.

Or maybe not. The amount of selenium in food depends on how much selenium is in the soil in which plants are grown or in the plants on which animals are fed. Many regions of Britain have low-selenium soil, which is why British wheat has low selenium. This means that some other food grown in Britain is lower in selenium than indicated in nutritional charts. But deficiency is a risk only for people whose food comes exclusively from a low-selenium region. Most people eat some foods from other countries and other regions of their own country. If most of your meat and vegetables come from a region with low-selenium soil, eating more fish and shellfish will help because fish get selenium from the marine ecosystem.

If you are concerned about your selenium status — if you live in a low-selenium region, eat mostly local food, and can't or won't eat seafood — you could turn to the richest source of it, namely, Brazil nuts. But no more than one nut per day! There is not only a recommended daily amount for selenium (55 mcg in the EU and the US) but also a tolerable upper limit (400 mcg) because it's toxic at high levels. Brazil nuts are so rich in selenium that just one nut per day provides roughly the whole of your daily amount, while five or six nuts takes you well over the tolerable upper limit. You won't suffer toxicity if you indulge in several Brazil nuts on the odd occasion, but consuming more than one Brazil nut per day over an extended period could be harmful. If you suspect that you have selenium deficiency, try eating one Brazil nut per day for two weeks and then cutting back to three or four per week (perhaps within a nut mixture). Those few Brazil nuts will meet a good proportion of your selenium requirement and you will get the rest from other foods.

By the way, governments in some countries with very low selenium have introduced measures to combat selenium deficiency in the population, such as importing foods from high-selenium countries or using selenium-enriched fertilizers. Selenium maps are available for some countries.

The bread-and-butter work of wheat

Here is a list of the types of dishes in which wheat (or rye or barley) is used and suggested ways of replacing them with quinoa, rice, or buckwheat.

Wheat-based dishes	Quinoa/rice/buckwheat alternatives
Carbohydrates in salads, e.g. cold pasta, couscous, croutons, the pastry in a quiche	Cooked, cold quinoa; cooked, cold rice pasta; savoury impossible pie (see the Recipes section)
Carbohydrates served with fish or meat, e.g. the pastry in pies	Cooked quinoa; rice; savoury impossible pie (see the Recipes section)
Soups or stews containing noodles, croutons, or pearl barley	Quinoa, either cooked with the dish or cooked separately and served on the top or on the side; buckwheat groats cooked with the dish
Couscous	Quinoa
Wheat pasta	Rice pasta
Wheat noodles	Rice noodles; soba (buckwheat noodles)
Wheat breakfast cereals	Gluten-free rice cereals; gluten-free buckwheat cereals; buckwheat porridge (see the Recipes section)
Wheat pancakes	Pancakes made with half-and-half rice flour and buckwheat flour
Wheat or rye sandwiches, wraps, toasties, etc.	Gluten-free equivalents made with a high proportion of rice flour and little or no tapioca starch
Wheat or multigrain crackers	Rice cakes; buckwheat crackers; quinoa and rice crackers
Cakes, cookies, etc.	Gluten-free equivalents made with a high proportion of rice flour and little or no tapioca starch
Pastry in desserts	Sweet impossible pie (see the Recipes section)
Semolina pudding	Ground rice pudding
Bread and butter pudding	Forget it

Additionally, you can continue with the familiar uses of rice, such as serving it with curries or stir-fries. Brown rice is better than white rice because it contains the bran layer and thus more fibre. However, it's OK to have white rice sometimes, for example, Arborio rice in risotto or short-grain rice in rice pudding.

New dietary staples

The preceding examination of the nutrients in, and uses of, wheat and alternative foods shows that no single food alone does the work of wheat. But you can replace wheat with a small set of foods — namely, quinoa, rice, and buckwheat. These are your new dietary staples. You don't have to eat all of them every day. Aim to have at least one of them every day and all of them during the course of a week.

If you find it difficult to work all three cereals into your weekly schedule, give preference to quinoa. However, it's best to include rice and buckwheat too because they have slightly different profiles of vitamins, minerals, and fibre. Moreover, the nutrition varies depending on whether you eat the grain or the flour or some other form. Therefore, if you eat all three of the new staples in various forms, it is more likely that you will cover all bases.

Brown rice grains are more nutritious than white rice grains, but white rice is also beneficial and you can use it if you find it easier to digest. However, the type of rice flour that works best in sauces or cakes is definitely brown.

If you previously used potatoes as a dietary staple, you can continue to eat them sometimes. Potatoes provide B vitamins, minerals, and fibre. However, they are higher in calories, a very high proportion of which comes from carbohydrates. So eat them in moderation, interspersing them with the new dietary staples.

Note that the new staples are not the only sources of the nutrients in wheat. A significant amount of B vitamins is found in meat and poultry, for example. The reason for the focus on quinoa, rice, and buckwheat is that they function as dietary staples in that you can eat one or more of them every day and obtain a significant proportion of your energy and nutrient needs from them. However, you also need to eat a variety of other foods during the course of each week to obtain the balance of your nutritional needs.

All the suggested new staples have a long shelf life. Consequently, you can reduce the cost by buying in bulk.

Alternative sets of staple foods are possible, but you would need a larger set of foods to get the same nutrition and versatility you get from quinoa, rice, and buckwheat. Furthermore, some of the other gluten-free cereals and pseudo-cereals are more expensive and less readily available.

Stuff that doesn't need replacing

Not all the substances in wheat need to be replaced. Some are bad for you and you'll be better off without them. The gluten, obviously. Possibly some other substances, whether naturally occurring or absorbed from a weed killer.

Similarly, not all the uses of wheat need to be replaced. The snacks eaten when not even hungry, for example. The bread rolls or naan bread eaten in a restaurant while waiting for the main course to arrive. Pizza. Until the late 1970s, pizza wasn't available in provincial England and people managed perfectly well without it; their weight was normal and they were nourished enough to be able to grow luscious, long hair.

Remedying common nutritional deficiencies

If you had celiac disease for many years before diagnosis (a common occurrence), your small intestine may have sustained a lot of damage. This damage can lead to malabsorption of iron, calcium, vitamin D, and folate. Many newly diagnosed celiacs are found to be mildly or seriously deficient in one or more of these nutrients. Mild deficiencies in these nutrients are also not uncommon in the general population.

Although healing of celiac intestinal damage begins quickly on a gluten-free diet, getting to the stage of absorbing significantly more of these nutrients from your food and replenishing your stores may take a few months. Meanwhile, you may temporarily need to take supplements. Your doctor should order blood tests to identify any deficiencies. Your doctor or dietitian may then recommend specific amounts of certain vitamins and/or minerals to get in your diet and/or in supplements. The blood tests should be repeated every few months until the results are normal and then followed up yearly.

Iron

Many newly diagnosed celiacs have a low level of iron, or even iron-deficiency anemia. Iron deficiency causes fatigue and pallor, and it should be corrected. If this applies to you, you will be advised to supplement your diet with iron until your level is normal. In the UK, you will probably be given an NHS prescription for iron tablets. There are two problems with this. First, iron tablets are available without prescription and it's cheaper to buy them over the counter than to pay the prescription charge. Second, the digestive side-effects of the tablets can be as unpleasant as the symptoms of celiac disease.

You can avoid the digestive side-effects by taking liquid iron instead. It's much easier to digest, though much more expensive. It tastes unpleasant, but if you drink it through a straw, you can get it down your throat without tasting it.

The best dietary source of iron is red meat because it contains the heme form of iron, which is well absorbed. White meat and fish are also good sources of heme iron. Some plant foods, including spinach, raisins, buckwheat, and quinoa, also contain iron but in the non-heme form, which is less well absorbed.

Vitamin C increases the absorption of non-heme iron. So, if you rely largely on foods containing non-heme iron or on supplements for your iron intake, have an orange or another good source of vitamin C at the same meal. Do not drink tea at the same meal because tannins decrease the absorption of non-heme iron.

Calcium and magnesium

Celiacs are at greater risk of osteoporosis due to malabsorption of calcium before diagnosis. If you have been diagnosed with celiac disease, your doctor should order a bone scan. If the scan shows that your bone density is below average, you will be advised to follow a calcium-rich diet or to take a calcium supplement, or both.

Dairy products are the best source of calcium. Sardines are also an excellent source; here, it's the bones that deliver the goods. Leafy green vegetables also contain calcium but in lesser amounts than dairy products. Of the leafy greens, kale is best (containing more calcium and being a good source of other nutrients) and spinach is worst (containing calcium but with low bioavailability).

Although the recommended daily intake of calcium is 800 mg in the EU, some dietitians advise celiacs to get 1000 mg per day, rising to 1200 mg per day for women over 50. To give you an idea of what this means, you could obtain about 1000 mg of calcium by eating all of the following during a day: a single-portion pot of yogurt, a matchbox-sized piece of hard cheese, a can of sardines, and a serving of kale. Or more cheese or milk instead of the sardines. Alternatively, you could obtain about 1000 mg of calcium from four 200 ml glasses of milk (not recommended, just to help you to visualize a quantity of calcium).

If you are lactose-intolerant, you need a plan for getting enough calcium because dairy products are indubitably the best sources of calcium in terms of both quantity and bioavailability, and most people get most of their calcium from dairy products. Your options are (1) get lactase tablets, which you can take when eating a lactose-containing meal, or (2) eat other calcium-containing foods, or (3) look for foods and drinks fortified with calcium, or (4) take a calcium supplement. Taking the lactase tablets is the easiest option. Eating enough of other calcium-containing foods to get the same amount of calcium as in a moderate amount of dairy products would involve eating an infeasibly large amount of leafy green vegetables. Fortified foods and drinks sound like a good option, except that many of them contain gluten. Calcium supplements are OK in the short term but not for long-term usage. Some combination of the four options might work. Many lactose-intolerant people actually produce small amounts of lactase and thus can consume small amounts of lactose without getting an adverse reaction. Some yogurt or a splash of milk in a hot drink might be OK.

Before you load up on calcium, ensure that you also get an adequate intake of magnesium because magnesium is needed for moving calcium from the blood into the bones, among many other important functions. Yet celiacs, especially women, are often advised to supplement with calcium and not advised to get more magnesium.

A blood test doesn't give a reliable indication of your magnesium level because less than 1% of it hangs out in the blood, the rest being stored in many types of cells throughout the body. So, rather than asking for a test, just be aware that magnesium deficiency is not uncommon in the general population and is more likely in celiacs due to malabsorption before diagnosis followed by reduced intake on the gluten-free diet if you're not careful. But you are careful, right? You do eat magnesium-rich foods such as buckwheat, leafy green vegetables, nuts, and seeds, right?

If you are advised to supplement with calcium, take a combined calcium and magnesium supplement and ensure that your total calcium-to-magnesium ratio from all sources does not exceed 2:1. Magnesium can also be absorbed through the skin. So an alternative way to boost your intake is to take baths with Epsom salt (magnesium sulphate) or Dead Sea salt (which additionally contains other minerals). Or occasionally rub a couple of squirts of magnesium oil into a couple of patches of skin after a shower.

Vitamin D and magnesium

Another nutrient important for bone health is Vitamin D, which helps to absorb calcium. Many other health benefits are claimed for vitamin D on the basis of interesting correlations, though some of these claims remain unproven. A deficiency of vitamin D is common in the general population and more likely in newly diagnosed celiacs because it's a fat-soluble vitamin, so absorption is reduced as a consequence of reduced fat absorption. There are three sources of vitamin D: food, UVB sunlight, and supplements.

The best food source is oily fish — salmon, mackerel, sardines, tuna, and herring. Egg yolks also provide some vitamin D. In some countries, some foods are fortified with vitamin D, for example, milk in the US and Canada. In the UK, it's mainly gluten-containing breakfast cereals and margarines that are fortified.

Noel Coward sang that only mad dogs and Englishmen go out in the midday sun. But Englishmen — and Englishwomen and anyone who lives in England — are justified in going out in the midday sun because there's only enough UVB sunlight in the UK to make vitamin D in April–September for two hours either side of midday. (Remember to adjust for British Summer Time; when the clock says midday, it's really only 11 am, which makes life harder for working people trying to make their lunch break coincide with the best time to get vitamin D.)

Sun exposure is safer than supplements from the perspective of vitamin D levels because overdosing on supplements can cause vitamin D toxicity, which cannot happen with sun exposure. Nonetheless, some people shun the sun completely due to fear of skin cancer. Yet you can get adequate vitamin D from sun exposure without burning and without increasing the risk of skin cancer. Here's how: go out with your face, hands, and arms uncovered for 10 minutes and then, if staying out, either cover up or apply sunscreen. Adjust the time depending on your skin colour; a dark-skinned person needs more sun exposure to get the same amount of vitamin D as a pale-skinned person. Also adjust to your local climate and follow local advice, especially in Australia, where the ozone layer is thinner.

In supplements, the active ingredient may be D_2 (ergocalciferol, a synthetic form) or D_3 (colecalciferol, the type naturally produced by the body after sun exposure). Supplements are available in the form of tablets or oral sprays. Tablets are absorbed by the digestive system. Oral sprays are absorbed through the blood vessels in the mouth.

Which of the three sources is best? The team from the BBC's "Trust Me, I'm a Doctor" TV programme did a small-scale experiment to test the effect of the three ways of getting vitamin D. Volunteer office workers were split into three groups. Group 1 went out in the sunshine for 10 minutes every day at lunchtime. Group 2 took a low-dose vitamin D supplement daily. Group 3 ate 100 g of oily fish three times a week. Vitamin D levels were measured before and after the 3-week experiment. The result was that vitamin D levels increased in all three groups by roughly the same amount.[14]

If you live in the northern hemisphere, you need a plan for maintaining a healthy level of vitamin D, even if you don't have celiac disease or have healed on the gluten-free diet. Vitamin D is stored in the liver. Your summer sunshine store might last through autumn (fall) but will be severely depleted by the end of winter if you don't actively do something about it. In winter, you must either eat oily fish two or three times a week (every week, without fail) or take a supplement. If you are unable or unwilling to expose your skin to the sun at any time of the year, follow either the fish regimen or the supplement regimen all year round.

As with calcium, so with vitamin D: before you load up on it, ensure that you also get an adequate intake of magnesium because magnesium is needed for converting vitamin D to its active form. If you take large doses of vitamin D when you have a low level of circulating magnesium, the body draws magnesium away from muscle tissue, which could cause muscular cramps. Yet celiacs are often advised to take vitamin D supplements without being advised to get more magnesium in their diet.

Folate and vitamin B12

Folate and vitamin B12 deficiencies are sometimes found in newly diagnosed celiacs, so the levels of these nutrients should be tested. It's particularly important to get your folate level tested if you are a celiac female planning to get pregnant because a deficiency increases the risk of neural tube defects in developing embryos.

Both folate and vitamin B12 are involved in making DNA, and each is involved in other essential functions. The symptoms of folate and B12 deficiency are similar (a form of anemia or other health problems). Don't try to diagnose these conditions yourself or to treat them with supplements because an excess of one of these nutrients can mask or worsen the symptoms of a deficiency of the other. If you are concerned about a possible deficiency of either of these nutrients, ask for a blood test and discuss the results with your doctor.

Folate is found in spinach, broccoli, avocados, bananas, quinoa, and buckwheat. B12 is found in meat, fish, shellfish, eggs, and dairy products.

If you are a gluten-free vegan, you need to be aware of two things: (1) vitamin B12 occurs naturally only in animal foods, and (2) the most common fortified foods are gluten-containing breakfast cereals and gluten-contaminated milk substitutes such as soy milk and oat milk. Consult a dietitian for personal advice about this.

Getting energised and repaired

Given that the main purpose of eating is to obtain energy, an important factor to consider when deciding on the broad composition of your diet is how to apportion your calorie intake between the energy-providing nutrients, which are fats, carbohydrates, and protein. These are called macronutrients because the required daily amounts are large (measured in grams rather than milligrams or micrograms).

The diet must include fats and protein. The clue is in the word "essential" in the phrases "essential fatty acids" and "essential amino acids". The diet should also include carbohydrates. Although it's technically possible to survive without carbohydrates, a diet with zero or very low carbohydrate is not advisable for any length of time because it may lead to nutritional deficiencies. However, most people would benefit from reducing the proportion of energy obtained from carbohydrates; more on this later.

Note that nature conveniently provides a mixture of the macronutrients in some foods. For example, beef contains protein and fat; chickpeas contain protein and carbohydrates; and milk and almonds contain protein, carbohydrates, and fats.

Protein

Although protein can provide energy, it is primarily needed for growth, repair, and maintenance. During digestion, proteins are broken down into their constituent amino acids. The amino acids are then available for producing the various types of proteins required by the body, according to the instructions encoded in the DNA in your cells. Examples are enzymes, antibodies, collagen in connective tissue, keratin in hair and skin, and proteins involved in muscle contraction.

(Incidentally, part of the gluten protein is the exception to the rule about protein digestion. The breakdown process gets as far as peptides, which are small chains of amino acids, but not as far as individual amino acids. This applies to everyone, with or without a gluten-related disorder. For most people, it's not a problem; the unusable peptides are simply excreted. In celiacs, a sequence of events leads to the peptides getting to places where they shouldn't be and setting off an autoimmune reaction.)

Excess amino acids cannot be stored in the body for long and are broken down and converted to glucose for energy. Because amino acids cannot be stored for long, a significant amount of protein must be in the diet every day.

The human body uses 20 amino acids. Some of these can be made in the body from other amino acids and thus don't have to be in the diet but the remainder must be in the diet because the body cannot make them. Foods that contain all the essential amino acids in the required proportions are called complete proteins. These are animal proteins — that is, meat, poultry, fish, milk, cheese, and eggs. Most of the plant sources of protein, such as peas, beans, nuts, seeds, and grains, are missing an adequate amount of one or more of the essential amino acids.

Recommendations for daily protein intake vary. Some say around 0.8 g of protein per kilogram of body weight. Some say 46–56 g per day. Some say 10% to 30% of total calorie intake. Men need more than women. Body builders need more again.

You can achieve one or more of the preceding recommendations if you build at least one meal a day around a good source of protein, such as meat or fish, and have either a smaller portion of a different meat or fish or another source of protein, such as cheese, eggs, or beans, at other meals or as snacks.

What are the implications of incomplete proteins for gluten-free vegetarians? By eating foods with complementary proteins, vegetarians can get an adequate protein intake. For example, peas contain lysine but limited methionine, whereas rice contains methionine but limited lysine. So if you eat rice with peas, you can get an adequate intake of both these essential amino acids. The same principle applies to some other combinations of legumes and cereals and to some combinations of legumes and nuts or seeds. The complementary proteins do not necessarily have to be eaten in the same meal but must be eaten within a 24-hour period. Of course, combining legumes and cereals is more difficult on the gluten-free diet because you have to avoid the gluten-containing cereals.

Fats and carbohydrates

To prevent the use of your protein intake for energy instead of repair and maintenance, you need a good intake of fats and carbohydrates. Consequently, the next decision is how to apportion your remaining calorie intake between fats and carbohydrates. The fat tide has recently turned, and, as Warren Buffett said, you only find out who is swimming naked when the tide goes out.

Dietary advice issued in the US in 1977 and in the UK in 1983 recommended reducing fat consumption to 30% of total energy intake and saturated fat to 10%, with the aim of reducing the incidence of coronary heart disease. In 2015, the *Open Heart* journal published a review of the evidence that was available at the time the advice was issued and found that the advice was not supported by the evidence. The reviewers, from the UK and the US, concluded that the advice should not have been introduced.[15] This news was well publicised and may be the first time that many members of the public became aware of doubts about official dietary advice. But doubts had been building up for some years, as recounted by Dr. Malcolm Kendrick in his book *The Cholesterol Con*.[16]

The findings of the 2015 review are truly shocking. When the low-fat dietary advice was issued, only six relevant trials of dietary interventions had looked at the relationship between dietary fat, serum cholesterol, and coronary heart disease. Five of these trials focused on secondary prevention in men who were already unhealthy rather than primary prevention in the general population. There was no difference in deaths from all causes between the treatment and comparison groups and no significant difference in deaths from coronary heart disease. Only one trial examined the consequence of a 10% saturated fat diet — and it reported a higher incidence of deaths from all causes and from coronary heart disease in the treatment group than in the comparison group. No women were included. No trial tested the dietary recommendations. No trial concluded that dietary recommendations should be drawn up. And there were methodological shortcomings.

Furthermore, no support was found for the idea that cholesterol has an intermediary role, that is, the idea that a high-fat diet leads to high cholesterol and that high cholesterol increases the risk of coronary heart disease. Although cholesterol levels were significantly reduced in the trials, this did not result in significant differences in deaths from coronary heart disease or all causes.

In my view, this is not surprising when you consider the functions of cholesterol. Its functions include the synthesis of the steroid hormones estrogen and testosterone and the synthesis of vitamin D (which is actually a steroid) when the skin is exposed to sunlight. Cholesterol also forms an essential part of the cell membranes of all cells in animals — including humans. That's why it is found in animal fat (meat, cheese, egg yolks). Given that the body is continuously making new cells, cholesterol is important. Because cholesterol is important, the body tries to conserve its supply. Most of the cholesterol circulating in your bloodstream is made in the liver and secreted into the blood from the bile. Only about 15% of cholesterol comes from diet. Much of the cholesterol is reabsorbed from the small intestine and recirculated.

(On a practical note, if your doctor has advised you to lower your cholesterol level, do ask whether your ratio of HDL or so-called "good cholesterol" to total cholesterol is good. Also be aware that there are two types of LDL or so-called "bad cholesterol" and only one of them furs up artery walls but blood tests don't distinguish between them. Also ask for an assessment of your overall risk of cardiovascular disease. If you are taking statins, do not stop taking them without consulting your doctor. As with the rest of this book, nothing in this section constitutes medical advice.)

There's another problem with the low-fat dietary advice, as pointed out in a 2014 editorial in *Open Heart* journal: the reduction in fat consumption led to a concomitant increase in carbohydrate consumption, paralleling an increase in the incidence of obesity and diabetes.[17] The same editorial pointed out that the condemnation of saturated fats led to guidelines recommending the replacement of saturated fats with polyunsaturated fats but without specifying which polyunsaturated fats. Yet increasing the amount of Omega-6 in the diet without increasing the amount of Omega-3 may increase the risk of coronary heart disease and overall mortality. Finally, the paper cites more recent research showing that a low-calorie, low-carbohydrate diet led to greater improvements in measurements of cardiovascular health than a low-calorie, low-fat diet.

A case study carried out by Damon Gameau on himself for the documentary *That Sugar Film* points to other health risks of a high-carb diet. Not having eaten refined sugar for nearly three years, Damon consumed the equivalent of 40 teaspoons of sugar a day (an amount that many Australians consume every day) for 60 days, under medical supervision. All the sugar was hidden in foods marketed as healthy, such as muesli bars and fruit juices; no confectionery, chocolate, or ice cream. During the study, he maintained his usual intake of 2,300 calories but with different proportions of fat and carbs. His usual diet had 50% of calories from fat, 26% from carbohydrates, and 24% from protein. During the study, he got 18% of calories from fat, 60% from carbohydrates, and 22% from protein. He became overweight and developed fatty liver disease within three weeks.

Because the low-fat dietary advice was largely unquestioned for decades, you will still come across recommendations to limit fat, especially saturated fat, in your diet and to obtain over half of your calories as carbohydrates. Even some recently refreshed guidelines repeat such advice. My understanding of the recent research (and also pre-1977 information) leads me to recommend tipping the balance in favour of fats, including saturated fats.

Not convinced to tip the balance because you know that each gram of carbohydrate contains four calories, whereas each gram of fat contains nine calories? Surely if one replaces a certain quantity of carbohydrate in one's diet with the same quantity of fat, the extra calories will lead to obesity? It's a good question. Even if you're underweight due to celiac disease and thus not currently worried about weight gain, you do need to consider this question. After a year or two of healing the gut on the gluten-free diet, celiacs become as prone to excess weight gain as the rest of the population. In other words, becoming overweight is possible but not inevitable. Fortunately, tipping the carbohydrate-to-fat balance in favour of fat does not make you fat because fats are digested and absorbed differently from carbohydrates.

The main dietary carbohydrates are sugars, starches, and fibre. Sugars comprise (1) simple sugars (monosaccharides), for example, glucose and fructose, (2) double sugars (two monosaccharides joined to make a disaccharide), for example, the sucrose in sugar cane and the lactose in milk sugar, and (3) polyols (sugar alcohols), such as sorbitol and xylitol. Some carbohydrates are more complex chemically, for example, the starch in potatoes and the cellulose in fruit and vegetable fibre. During digestion, double sugars and starches are broken down into glucose, which can be immediately circulated in the bloodstream to cells all over the body and then used to generate energy in the cells. If the glucose is not immediately needed for energy, it is converted to glycogen and stored in the liver and skeletal muscles. Stored glycogen provides an energy reserve, which is converted back to glucose when needed (between meals). If the energy reserves are replete, any excess is converted to fat and stored as body fat.

In contrast, fats and oils are triglycerides. (Oils are simply fats that are liquid at room temperature.) During digestion, triglycerides are broken down into three fatty acids and glycerol. (Saturated and unsaturated fats differ in the type of chemical bonds between the fatty acids.) After traversing some more metabolic pathways, the components of fats can be used to generate cellular energy, and any excess is stored as body fat.

So you can get energy from either fats or carbohydrates, and you can get body fat from either source. But the differences in digestion and metabolism mean that fats release energy slowly, whereas carbohydrates supply energy quickly by raising the level of blood glucose. This applies especially to simple sugars but also to complex carbohydrates to a lesser extent. Glucose cannot safely be left in the blood for long, so a quick rise in blood glucose results in a spike in the level of the hormone responsible for pulling excess glucose from the blood and sending it on its way — insulin. Over time, insulin spikes can lead to insulin resistance, type 2 diabetes, and obesity. These spikes can also result in energy peaks and troughs. You may feel hungry again soon after eating a sugary meal and then be tempted to have a snack — which will probably contain more sugar, resulting in another peak and another trough, and so on. By contrast, fats do not affect blood glucose. They release energy at a steadier rate over a longer period. They also make you feel full for longer, so you will be less likely to want to snack.

If you are eating a lot of carbohydrates, it is advisable to replace some of them with fats. When you do eat carbohydrates, combine them with fats. Eating fat in the same meal as carbohydrates decreases the rate at which the sugar in the carbohydrates is released.

Note that the aim is to change the balance of carbs and fats, *not* to add fats to your existing carbs. If you have a cheese omelette for breakfast, skip the (gluten-free) toast or cereal. If you snack on nuts and seeds, have them instead of, not in addition to, some confectionery. If you add cream or cheese to a pasta sauce, serve it with less pasta. On some days, have your main meal without any potato, pasta, rice, or other carbs. You will find that a steak (complete with the fat layer) served with carrots and a steamed green vegetable will provide enough energy to power you until the next meal. Or a piece of fish with stir-fried vegetables and pine nuts or cashews. It's especially good to skip the carbs at dinner on a day when you've succumbed to a slice of gluten-free cake earlier in the day.

You might think that your diet already has enough fat because you never bought the low-fat message or low-fat varieties of foods and drinks. But if you've been around since the 1970s or 1980s, you have probably reduced your fat intake since then without realizing it because many manufacturers and restaurateurs reduced the fat in their regular products and meals. Out went thick natural yogurts, in came runny fruity yogurts with added sugar. Out went full-fat milk, in came skimmed milk. Out went spaghetti carbonara, in came stuffed peppers. Out went cuts of meat complete with fat, in came lean cuts and reduced-fat minced meat. Out went sour varieties of apples, in came sweet varieties. Somewhere along the line, you may have stopped putting a knob of butter on your vegetables, stinted on the amount of butter on toast, stopped pouring cream over fruit salad, and stopped filling sticks of celery with original full-fat Philadelphia cheese. Consequently, following a higher-fat diet may take a conscious effort.

We started considering the question of how to split calories between fats and carbs on the assumption that your protein intake is already appropriate. If your diet has actually been protein-deficient until now, you could replace some of your carbohydrates with protein. Protein has little effect on blood glucose levels and, like fat, leaves you feeling fuller for longer and decreases the rate at which sugar is released.

In the following sections, we'll look at which types of fats and carbohydrates to favour and which to avoid.

Omega oils and other polyunsaturated fats

As already mentioned, dietary guidelines issued in the 1970s and 1980s recommended the replacement of saturated fats with polyunsaturated fats but without specifying which polyunsaturated fats. There should have been guidance on the balance between Omega-3 and Omega-6.

Most of the polyunsaturated fatty acids can be made in the body from other fats and other nutrients, except Omega-3 and Omega-6 essential fatty acids. They are called "essential" because they are needed for specific functions (not just for energy) but cannot be made from other nutrients and thus must be in the diet. It's important to get the right *balance* of Omega-3 and Omega-6 and the right *type* of Omega-3.

Omega-3 oils and Omega-6 oils compete for certain enzymes on certain metabolic pathways, so the ratio between them is important. Opinions on the optimal ratio vary, but it is generally agreed that Western diets have too much Omega-6 and not enough Omega-3. Basically, Omega-6 is pro-inflammatory, whereas Omega-3 is anti-inflammatory. Therefore, it's good to have Omega-3 in the diet to prevent diseases involving inflammation. You do need Omega-6 too because some inflammation is normal when responding to an infection or injury and because, well, it's essential. But you can get enough Omega-6 without trying.

To get a good ratio of Omega-3 to Omega-6 in your diet, you need to eat foods with much more Omega-3 than Omega-6 and to limit foods with much more Omega-6 than Omega-3.

Good foods from this perspective are oily fish — mackerel, salmon, trout, sardines, tuna, and herring. White fish such as cod and haddock also contain more Omega-3 than Omega-6, though not as much Omega-3 as the oily fish. Flaxseeds (also called linseeds) have a good balance of Omega-3 to Omega-6, but it's a different type of Omega-3 to that found in fish and not as useful (more on this soon).

Bad foods from this perspective include sunflower oil, soybean oil, corn oil, and palm oil. Note that, if you are trying to improve your 3-to-6 balance, it makes no sense to eat canned mackerel in sunflower oil; the benefit of the Omega-3 in the fish is negated by the Omega-6 in the sunflower oil.

As well as improving your 3-to-6 balance, you also need to get the right type of Omega-3 fatty acids; they are not all biochemically equal. Eicosapentaenoic acid (EPA) and docosahexaenoic acid (DHA) are the most useful for health. EPA and DHA together improve cardiovascular health and help to prevent or control inflammatory diseases. DHA additionally helps to maintain normal vision and brain function. EPA and DHA are found in oily fish. The fish get the oil from algae they eat (or from smaller fish that have eaten algae), so an alternative source is algal oil.

Alpha-linolenic acid (ALA) is another Omega-3. This is found in flaxseed oil, walnuts, and some green vegetables. Although the body can convert ALA to EPA and DHA, only very low amounts are converted, most ALA being used simply for energy. This means that, although plant sources of Omega-3 help with the overall balance between Omega-3 and Omega-6, they cannot substitute for oily fish in the diet.

Saturated and monounsaturated fats

As well as polyunsaturated fats, you also need saturated and monounsaturated fats. One reason is that you need fats that you can safely use for cooking. When sunflower oil and other oils high in polyunsaturated fat are heated, they oxidize and produce high quantities of aldehydes, according to research done at De Montfort University.[18]. Aldehydes are chemicals linked with heart disease and cancer. Saturated fats produce the lowest amount of harmful chemicals when heated. Therefore, frying and roasting is best done in butter, lard, goose fat, duck fat, or coconut oil.

Oils with a high proportion of monounsaturated fats, such as olive oil and rapeseed oil (canola oil), are in between polyunsaturated oils and saturated fats in terms of aldehydes produced under heat. Therefore, they may be used for some frying.

Saturated and monounsaturated fats also provide other benefits. As already mentioned, saturated fats are not the bad guys they have been portrayed as. They provide energy and make you feel fuller for longer, thus reducing reliance on carbohydrates. Monounsaturated fats kept their reputations as good guys throughout controversies about total fat intake, as it is believed that they are good for heart health. Sources of monounsaturated fats are olive oil, avocados, some nuts (including almonds and hazelnuts), and some seeds.

Complex carbohydrates

For the carbohydrate part of your diet, give preference to foods that contain starch and/or fibre. In particular, go for vegetables, beans, potatoes, sweet potatoes, and gluten-free whole grains such as brown rice, quinoa, and gluten-free oats. Unlike sugary carbs, these foods provide a good quantity of vitamins and minerals and are good for digestion.

Sugars

Limit daily added sugars to the equivalent of 6 teaspoons (women) or 9 teaspoons (men). This advice applies to everyone, not only to fat people. There are many skinny fat people — people who look slim and have little subcutaneous fat (visible fat under the skin) but lots of visceral fat (invisible fat around the internal organs) and thus a high body fat percentage. If you're young and have a low body fat percentage despite having a sweet tooth, you might think that you're getting away with it. But if you continue to overindulge a sweet tooth, the sugar hobgoblin will probably catch up with you later, displacing the sugar plum fairy.

There are two types of sugars: naturally occurring sugars and free sugars. Naturally occurring sugars are found in fresh fruit and vegetables and in milk. All these foods are good for you. They are all good sources of vitamins and minerals, and they're not too sweet. Furthermore, the fibre in fruit and vegetables slows the digestion of the sugars in them, thus preventing insulin spikes.

Free sugars, as defined by the World Health Organization (WHO), are "monosaccharides and disaccharides added to foods and beverages by the manufacturer, cook or consumer, and sugars naturally present in honey, syrups, fruit juices and fruit juice concentrates". Glucose and fructose are monosaccharides. Sucrose (table sugar, or refined sugar) is a disaccharide, half glucose and half fructose. The WHO recommends reducing the intake of free sugars to less than 10% of total energy intake for general health benefits and suggests a further reduction to below 5% for additional dental health benefits.[19] On a 2,000 calorie diet (a common recommendation for women), 5% of energy intake is roughly 25 g (6 teaspoons). Free sugars are also known as added sugars.

One problem with simple sugars is that they do not provide vitamins, minerals, or fibre. This is why they are called "empty calories". Another problem is their link with obesity and the consequent increased risk of type 2 diabetes.

Some scientists believe that fructose is more harmful to health than glucose, though some scientists disagree. It's possible that fructose negatively affects only people who aren't very active and who consume it to excess. Unfortunately, excess consumption has become more common in recent decades. Traditionally, there was little fructose in our diets and most of it came in whole fruit. Now, fructose is added to many processed foods and drinks and most of it comes from refined sugar (sucrose) and high-fructose corn syrup.

To cut down on free sugars, it is necessary to look out for hidden sugars. Free sugars may be hidden in two senses.

First, free sugars are added not only to sweet-tasting confections such as cakes, biscuits, and desserts but also to many foods perceived as savoury — for example, pasta sauces, ketchup, chutney, low-fat yogurt, ready meals, and muesli bars. Free sugars are also added to many soft drinks, including some perceived as healthy, such as flavoured mineral waters. They are even added to some products marketed for weight loss!

Second, checking for added sugars on food labels is even more difficult than checking for gluten. When I first heard the phrase "hidden sugars", I thought that many people were simply not reading labels. Surely if they looked, they would find? Then I realized that some added sugars are almost as well hidden as the plans for the destruction of planet Earth in *The Hitch Hiker's Guide to the Galaxy*; the information might as well be in the planning department in Alpha Centauri.

Nutrition declarations in many countries indicate the total carbohydrate and how much of that total consists of sugars. "Sugars" in this context means *all* monosaccharides and disaccharides. Manufacturers are not required to distinguish between naturally occurring monosaccharides and disaccharides and added ones. Some products without added sugar have more sugars in total than some products containing cane sugar or glucose syrup. A relatively high level of sugars may be fine if the sugars come from fruits, vegetables, or milk. But labels don't tell you where the sugars come from. Even if you have thought to check the label of an apparently savoury product for sugars and confirmed the presence of added sugars, you still don't know what percentage of the total sugars they constitute. If no free sugars have been added to a product, the manufacturer may put "no added sugar" on the label. In the absence of such a statement, the best you can do is to look for clues in the ingredients list.

Because ingredients are listed in descending order of weight, you might try to glean information from the ordering. However, the ordering still leaves a big information gap. For example, if a product has three ingredients, it could be that the first ingredient constitutes 90% of the product, the second 8%, and the third 2%. Or it could be that the first two ingredients constitute 45% each and the third 10%. So, if the first ingredient is dates and the second ingredient is glucose-fructose syrup, some of the sugars come from the dates and some from the syrup. In the first example, the syrup would be 8% of the product. In the second example, it would be 45%. To add to the confusion, an added sugar may be hidden within another ingredient such as apple juice concentrate or strawberry jam.

"Sugar" in the ingredients list means sucrose. Other names for added sugars include cane sugar and beet sugar (along with their "organic", "raw", and "brown" counterparts), invert sugar, molasses, caramel, glucose syrup, and agave syrup. In the US, you will often see high-fructose corn syrup. In the EU, the usage of this syrup is lower and it's called glucose-fructose syrup or fructose-glucose syrup.

If you find it difficult to cut down on sugar due to its addictive properties, try cutting it out completely for at least two weeks. In the first few days, you might have withdrawal symptoms such as brain fog. Then the symptoms will abate and you will no longer crave sugar. If you decide to reintroduce some sugar after at least two sugar-free weeks, you will find that your palate has been reconditioned. Very sugary foods will taste too sweet, making it easier to stay within the recommended limit.

By the way, many products proclaimed as sugar-free contain artificial sweeteners instead. Although sweeteners have no calories, their sweet taste fools your body into reacting as if you had eaten sugar — that is, releasing insulin and going into fat storage mode. It is also suspected that sweeteners adversely affect the control of appetite.

Energy balance: food portions and exercise portions

Energy levels and body weight do not depend solely on the difference between calorie intake and calorie expenditure; the calories in fats act differently in the body from the calories in carbohydrates, and added sugars act differently from complex carbohydrates. Nonetheless, weight is largely determined by the balance between total calorie intake and expenditure; eating 3,000 calories while sitting on a couch all day would be bad, regardless of the source of the calories.

So, should you count calories? Calorie-counting is a bore and not helpful for most people most of the time. If your weight is normal and stable (apart from being a little higher in winter), there's no point in counting calories. But if you are overweight or underweight or if you are unintentionally gaining or losing weight when you don't need to, you might countenance counting.

Here's a thought: if you frequently eat with another adult of the opposite sex and the amount of food on each plate is usually the same, it's possible that one of you is overeating or one of you is under-eating.

On the other side of the energy equation, there's exercise. Just as you are mindful of portion size when it comes to food, so you should consider exercise in terms of portion size; get the right amount of it. Official recommendations in the UK and the US are:

- At least 150 minutes a week of moderate aerobic activity (equal to 30 minutes a day on 5 days a week) *or* 75 minutes a week of vigorous aerobic activity, *and*
- Strength training exercises at least twice a week.

Note the phrase "at least" in these recommendations. Many exercise experts advocate a greater amount of exercise, especially for anyone who is overweight or who wants to boost athletic performance.

Moderate aerobic activities include mowing the lawn, fast walking, and volleyball. Vigorous aerobic activities include aerobics classes, running, and football. For strength training, you can use weights, resistance bands, or exercises that use your own body weight such as push-ups. Other activities that work all the major muscles, like heavy gardening, also count toward your strength training quota.

The official exercise recommendations are aimed primarily at preventing heart disease. Many celiacs are more concerned about prevention or management of osteoporosis. For this purpose, you additionally need to do activities for improving the sense of balance. It's well known that people with osteoporosis are more likely to fracture a bone if they fall. But why do they fall? Sometimes, it's due to a poor sense of balance.

How is your sense of balance now? How long can you stand on one leg? For people with normal mobility, one minute is normal and anything less than 30 seconds is a concern. How long does it take you to get up out of a chair, walk three metres (10 feet), turn around, and sit down again? For people with normal mobility, a normal result is 10 seconds or less. If your balance is not normal, try to improve it, so as to reduce your risk of falls. Strength training exercises are helpful because they improve muscle mass, but you also need exercises specifically aimed at improving balance. If you are concerned about your sense of balance, consult a physical therapist for a more precise assessment and for specific exercises.

Your food and exercise portions need to be reviewed periodically. After middle age, your daily calorie requirement goes down. To minimize middle-aged spread, you must either eat less or exercise more, or both. Eating less requires even more focus on healthy eating; foods with empty calories must be avoided in order to ensure that you still get an adequate amount of vitamins and minerals while eating less. Exercising more not only burns calories but also provides additional benefits, such as helping to prevent osteoporosis and other age-related diseases, improving posture, and getting an exercise high.

Supporting physical and mental health

Food not only supplies energy but also supports physiological functions and helps to maintain physical and mental health. This is where vitamins, minerals, and phytonutrients come in. Most of these are considered micronutrients because the required daily amounts are small (measured in milligrams or micrograms rather than grams). Fibre and so-called "good bacteria" also support good health.

Vitamins

Vitamins are organic substances that are essential for biochemical processes, including the activity of neurotransmitters and hormones, the expression of genes, the creation of bone and connective tissue, wound healing, blood clotting, vision, and the absorption of other nutrients.

Some vitamins are fat-soluble, whereas others are water-soluble.

The fat-soluble vitamins are A, D, E, and K. They are found in fatty and oily foods, including oily fish, milk, butter, seed oils, and liver. They are also found in orange vegetables and leafy green vegetables. If you get more fat-soluble vitamins than you need on a given day, they are stored in the liver and fatty tissue. (Other animals do likewise, which is why liver is a good source of these vitamins.) If you get less of these vitamins than you need on a given day, your body obtains the shortfall from its stores.

The water-soluble vitamins are the B vitamins, folate, and vitamin C. The B vitamins are found mainly in vegetables, grains, and meat. Vitamin C is found mainly in citrus fruits (oranges, lemons, limes, grapefruit), tomatoes, potatoes, and sweet potatoes. If you get more of these vitamins than you need on a given day, they are excreted in the urine rather than stored. So they should be in your diet every day.

Minerals

Minerals are inorganic substances that collectively support many functions, including building bones and teeth, controlling fluid balance, transmitting nerve impulses, making proteins, and metabolism. Over a dozen minerals are believed to be essential, but only iron and calcium are needed in appreciable amounts. The rest are needed only in small amounts, some only in trace amounts.

Some minerals are electrolytes — that is, compounds that dissociate into positive and negative ions when dissolved in body fluids and can conduct electricity. Four particular minerals are important for the electrical activity of neurons and muscle cells – sodium, potassium, magnesium, and calcium. Have you ever suffered from diarrhea (and thus fluid loss) to the extent of feeling completely wiped out and then taken a medicine that replaces the lost electrolytes and rapidly recovered a sense of wellbeing? If so, you know the importance of electrolytes.

The ratio of potassium to sodium is important. Sodium increases blood pressure, whereas potassium lowers it by promoting the excretion of sodium in the urine. Many people consume too much sodium (as sodium chloride, in salt). Therefore, it's important to eat potassium-rich foods to redress the balance.

Calcium is important not only as an electrolyte but also for bone health. But the ratio of calcium to magnesium should not exceed 2:1. Therefore, it's important to include some magnesium-rich foods in your diet.

Fortunately, many magnesium-rich foods are also rich in potassium. These foods include bananas, pumpkin seeds, dark chocolate, buckwheat, and spinach.

Phytonutrients

Phytochemicals, also known as phytonutrients, are compounds in plants that provide some health benefits. Here is a small selection of phytochemicals from the major groups, along with some claimed health benefits and some good dietary sources.

- Polyphenols.
  - Anthocyanin. Slowing the progression of glaucoma, antioxidant, anti-cancer, anti-inflammatory. Blueberries, bilberries, blackcurrants, black grapes, aubergines (eggplant).
  - Catechins. Lowering blood pressure, antioxidant. Cocoa, green tea.
- Carotenoids.
  - Lutein. Reducing the risk of macular degeneration and cataracts. Kale, spinach, broccoli, romaine lettuce, watercress, eggs.
  - Lycopene. Protection against prostate and ovarian cancer, protection against UV-induced skin damage, maintenance of normal cardiovascular function, other benefits too numerous to mention. Tomato paste, tomatoes, watermelon.
- Glucosinolates. Protection against cancer, good for cardiovascular health. Brussels sprouts, cabbage, broccoli.
- Stanols and sterols. Lowering cholesterol. No fresh food with significant amounts but available in "functional foods" — that is, food products to which compounds with specific health benefits have been added.

Beware the hype about phytonutrients. There is insufficient evidence for many of the health claims to count them as scientifically proven. Lycopene is a prime example. Many claims have been made for it, but evidence-based reviews have concluded that no cause and effect relationship has been established between consumption of lycopene and some of the claimed benefits. Furthermore, you might find it difficult to eat the amount of tomatoes or tomato paste necessary to get any potential benefit. Eat tomatoes anyway because they contain many vitamins and minerals in addition to lycopene and are easy to grow, even on a balcony. Just don't expect a tomato habit to be a panacea for all ills.

Fibre

Fibre is a concern for people on a gluten-free diet because many processed gluten-free foods provide less fibre than wheat-based equivalents and fibre is needed for good digestion and colon health and more besides. However, many naturally gluten-free foods contain fibre and you should be eating them anyway as part of a balanced diet.

Fibre has been loosely classified into two types. *Soluble* fibre *slows* digestion by attracting water to itself and forming a gel. It beneficially affects the absorption of glucose and fats. It also ferments in the gut, increasing intestinal gas. *Insoluble* fibre *speeds* the movement of food and waste along the digestive tract, keeping you regular. It also alleviates constipation by increasing stool bulk.

I mentioned the two types because many people who go gluten-free are motivated to do so by digestive problems, one way or the other. However, some scientists want to eliminate the distinction between soluble and insoluble fibre, on the basis that not all soluble fibre affects absorption and some insoluble fibre ferments. Furthermore, the effects can vary from person to person. Many fibrous foods contain both types anyway. So, for good general health, simply eat foods that contain both types of fibre.

Some good gluten-free sources of the various loosely-defined types of fibre are as follows.

- Insoluble: dates and the skins of potatoes and tomatoes
- Soluble: oats, peas, beans, and lentils
- Both types: quinoa, buckwheat, pumpkin seeds, broccoli, cabbage, carrots, celery, cucumber, kale, raisins, and apples and plums (soluble on the inside, insoluble in the skins)

Many other vegetables and fruits contain both types of fibre. So eat them — not only for the fibre but also for the vitamins and minerals.

Good bacteria

Your body plays host to lots of microorganisms, mainly bacteria, residing mainly in the gut and the skin. How does your microbiome — the population of microorganisms in your body — affect your health and what can you do about it? This is an area of active research and there are tantalizing suggestions that practical applications for human health may become available, but our current knowledge is limited.

However, three things can already be stated with certainty. First, the good bacteria help to digest and absorb some nutrients, prevent the growth of bad bacteria, and develop the immune system. Second, lack of good bacteria and lack of diversity among them are correlated with various diseases, including inflammatory bowel conditions, type 2 diabetes, obesity, and depression. Third, the population of bacteria can be changed through diet. Dietary approaches include probiotics and prebiotics.

Probiotic foods contain good bacteria, for example, live yogurt containing bifidobacterium and lactobacillus acidophilus.

Prebiotics are fibre compounds that act as food for good bacteria, mainly inulin and fructo-oligosaccharide. High amounts of prebiotics are found in chicory root, garlic, leeks, onions, and asparagus. A lesser amount is found in unripe bananas. Note that inulin is sometimes added to processed foods, and this is one circumstance where processing can be advantageous. The manufacturer's motivation may or may not be good; inulin is increasingly used to replace sugar and/or fat and/or flour because it delivers a slightly sweet taste and creamy texture, enabling manufacturers to market their products as low-sugar and/or low-fat and/or gluten-free while retaining the "moreish" factor. You can have too much of a good thing; while inulin can improve digestive health, it can cause digestive discomfort in some people, especially if large amounts are introduced into the diet suddenly.

Oiling the wheels of nutritional savviness

Traffic lights and olive oil: nutrition declarations

While you're reading food labels to check for gluten, you might as well take the opportunity to check the nutrition declaration. Maybe you won't immediately do anything with that information. But after a while, you might notice patterns in the information and develop a sense of what quantities of what nutrients should be expected in given types of food products.

The regulations regarding nutrition information on food labels vary from country to country and from time to time. Additionally, the recommended amounts of specific nutrients change from time to time, as new scientific opinions are adopted. However, there are some commonalities across space and time.

The nutrition declaration includes a nutrient if it is present in a significant amount and if a recommended amount has been defined. The amount is expressed as a percentage of a reference intake or per 100 g /100 ml or per specified serving size. Although reference intakes vary by age and gender, only one value is used on food labels. In the EU, the reference intake is the average daily amount that meets the requirements of 97.5 % of the adult population and it is called the RDA (recommended daily amount). In the US and Canada, the reference intake (RDI) is used to determine the Daily Value (DV), which is used for nutrition labelling.

If nutrient amounts are expressed per serving size, check whether the specified size bears any resemblance to what you actually serve to yourself.

Regarding salt, the EU Food Information to Consumers regulation requires that nutritional declarations show the amount of salt, not the amount of the sodium constituent. If labels in your neck of the woods declare an amount of sodium, multiply that by 2.5 to get the amount of salt.

Calories are indicated in either kilocalories (kcal) or kilojoules (kJ). The term "kilocalorie" is used interchangeably with "calorie"; 1,000 calories is written as 1,000 kcal. To convert from kcal to kJ, multiply by 4.2.

In the EU, the Food Information for Consumers regulation permits member states to recommend the use of additional forms of expression or presentation of the nutrition declaration, provided no obstacle to the free movement of goods within the EU is created. Under this regulation, while still an EU member, the UK introduced a front-of-pack nutrition label including colour coding (traffic light colours of red, amber, and green) for total fat, saturated fats, sugars, and salt. Provision of this label in the UK is voluntary and some large multinationals have chosen not to use it.

The European Commission launched an investigation into whether the British traffic light presentation impedes trade between EU countries, following complaints from southern European member states that it's simplistic and doesn't distinguish between junk food and foods naturally high in fat. Italians say that their cheese, ham, and olive oil are classified as red due to high fat content, even though such foods are used in traditional Mediterranean cuisine as part of a balanced diet. I'm with the Italians on this; these foods are indeed part of a balanced diet. The Commission formally asked the UK authorities to respond to the complaint in October 2014. This is the first stage of infringement proceedings. The UK submitted its response in December 2014. The Commission subsequently had meetings with both sides but, as at mid-2019, had not decided on the next steps. Lack of progress seems unrelated to the UK's exit from the EU, rather due to other EU member states being divided on the issue, with some joining in with the original complainants and others deciding to introduce their own traffic light labels.

Anyway, it's better to read the full list of ingredients and the mandatory nutrition declaration on the back of the pack. Otherwise, you could buy a low-salt, low-sugar product on the basis of green lights on the front, only to read the back when you get home and find lots of artificial colours and flavourings but few vitamins and minerals. Furthermore, the traffic light system still considers saturated fat to be a bad thing.

Gluten freedom and low-grade oil: ingredients lists

Don't focus on "gluten-free" to the exclusion of "goodness full". The front of a pack may proclaim that the product inside contains no gluten, no dairy products, no nuts, and no sugar but not what it *does* contain. It's important to look at the list of ingredients on the back, especially if the excluded ingredients would normally be in the relevant type of product. If the ingredients list consists mostly of low-grade oils, artificial flavourings, sweeteners, tapioca starch, and a long list of chemicals, it's not part of a healthy diet. Look for gluten-free *and* good.

Luxury and coconut oil: front-of-pack marketing messages

The front of the pack is for the marketing messages, and these messages start with the product name. Look out for bamboozling product names like Beatific Beetroot Soup, Salary-Increasing Salad Dressing, Stratospheric Strudel, and Yeswikan Nut Bar. I made these up. But they're not dissimilar to real product names. In fact, I had to reject some of my made-up silly names because they turned out to be the names of real products. You're supposed to think that, if you buy the product, you will acquire the named characteristic. The marketing people do not explicitly claim that this will happen. They imply it and hope that you will infer it.

The marketing messages continue with slogans. Egg boxes provide a rich source of examples. You may see "barn eggs", "farm fresh", "local", "natural", or the name of a posh-sounding farm. In the absence of "free range", these slogans are all ways of distracting your attention from the fact that the eggs are *not* from free-range chickens. Think about it. Suppliers always want to make the boldest claims that they can legally make. If they have gone to the extra time and expense entailed in producing free-range eggs, why would they not put "free range" on the box? Why would they put "farm fresh" instead? The suppliers of "farm fresh" eggs and suchlike have not explicitly claimed that the eggs are produced in accordance with best animal welfare practices or that they are better for you than any other eggs. They imply it and hope that you will infer it.

Package designers may also use vague adjectives and different font sizes to emphasize a positive message and de-emphasize other information. The producer of a sachet of hot chocolate mix has got this down to a fine art. The front of the pack carries the Fairtrade logo and proclaims "Luxury Hot Chocolate" in a large font size, with "Luxury" in italics — followed by "Flavoured Drink" in a much smaller font size. On the back of the pack, the ingredients list is as follows.

"sugar, **whey** powder, fat reduced cocoa powder (11%), glucose syrup, hydrogenated coconut oil, **milk** proteins, salt, anti-caking agent E341, stabiliser E340, emulsifier E471, flavouring"

The nutrition declaration gives sugar as 69.2 g per 100 g, and the producer has inadvertently made it easier to estimate how much of that sugar is added rather than naturally occurring. We already know that sugar is the main ingredient and that the cocoa powder comprises only 11% of the product (even though it's the only chocolatey ingredient in a luxury chocolate mix). Because the product is Fairtrade-certified, the label reveals that it's the cocoa and sugar that are fair-traded and that these total 54.7% of the product. Therefore, the sugar ingredient comprises 43.7% of the product. The glucose syrup, coming after the cocoa powder in the list, could comprise as much as 10% of the product. By adding that to the "sugar", we can conclude that the product could contain up to 53% added sugars.

The next thing to note is that when "coconut oil" is transmuted into "hydrogenated coconut oil", it is changed from a healthy fat into an unhealthy trans fat.

You wouldn't know any of this if you relied on the messages on the front of the pack, which heavily emphasize "luxury" and "Fairtrade". The meaning of "luxury" is vague in this context. "Fairtrade" does have a definite meaning; it means that the farmers and plantation workers are paid a fair price and have decent working conditions, which is obviously good for the workers. The marketing people do not explicitly claim that luxury products containing fair-traded crops are good for you. They imply it and hope that you will infer it.

I have also seen a marketing message implying goodness on a packet of crisps, but I took that with a pinch of salt.

Investigative journalists sometimes run stories exposing the fact that particular popular foods or drinks contain very high amounts of sugar or salt, even though they are perceived as healthy choices by the average consumer. The main reason that average consumers don't already know that the products in question are unhealthy is that they make inferences from the marketing messages on the front of the pack instead of reading the regulated information on the back of the pack. Or they get takeaway food or drink without asking what's in it. Fortunately, you are not an average consumer. You are above average. Nonetheless, let's hope that these stories keep coming, so that everyone is better informed.

Vitamins and fish oil: food supplements

If your blood test results are normal and you have not been advised to take supplements by a doctor or a dietitian, it's better to try to stay healthy by eating a healthy diet rather than by routinely taking supplements, for the following reasons.

- Some nutrients are *not as effective* when taken in supplemental form as when absorbed from food.

- A supplement may supply *too much* of the active ingredients, resulting in so-called "expensive urine"; B vitamins, for example, cannot be stored for future use and any excess is excreted.

- A supplement may supply *way too much* of the active ingredients, resulting in toxicity; it's possible to overdose on some nutrients when you take them as supplements but not when you get them in food (or through sun exposure, in the case of vitamin D).

- A supplement may supply *too little* of the active ingredients due to the use of chemical forms with low bioavailability. A supplement can claim to contain 40% of the recommended daily amount of a given nutrient even if it's in a form that's only 2% bioavailable and thus actually provides only 0.8% of the daily amount. In general, organic compounds are more bioavailable than inorganic compounds. In general, you get what you pay for; highly bioavailable ingredients are more likely to be found in the more expensive brands than in the cheap brands.

- A supplement may supply *too little* of the active ingredients due to many vitamins and minerals being packed into one tablet. Some single-nutrient tablets have to be fairly large in order to carry a significant percentage of the recommended daily amount. Yet a multivitamin tablet has to carry many nutrients in the same space. This is likely to be particularly problematic for one-a-day multivitamin tablets.

- Supplementation can result in *mineral imbalances*. For example, too much zinc can inhibit the absorption of copper.

- Some supplements *harm your health* when taken regularly over a long period. For example, supplementing with vitamins A or E increases the risk of early death,[20] supplementing with vitamin E increases the risk of lung cancer,[21] and supplementation with calcium is linked to a greater risk of kidney stones[22] and plaque buildup in arteries.[23]

- Some supplements *interact with medicines*, either intensifying or weakening their effects. If you are on any medication, do not take supplements without first consulting your doctor.

- Supplements may *harm your financial health*.

There are a few exceptions to the general rule of avoiding supplements, as follows.

- If you don't expose your skin to the sun or eat oily fish, take a vitamin D supplement.

- If you don't eat oily fish, and especially if you have an inflammatory disease, consider taking a supplement containing Omega-3 EPA + DHA — either fish oil or algal oil. If you can't easily digest gel capsules, try bottled oil.

- If you have a poor diet for reasons beyond your control (for example, if you depend on institutional catering) or if you are recovering from a serious disease or struggling to keep healthy as you age, consider taking a good multivitamin and multimineral supplement.

Apricot kernels and snake oil: health claims

Many countries have regulations regarding health claims about food substances on labels. The general principles and the specific permitted claims vary from country to country, being markedly different in the US, the EU, and Japan. Furthermore, the situation changes whenever applications for approval of health claims are evaluated or contested, which makes it hard to keep up with the state of the art, let alone the state of the science. Fortunately, most food businesses won't risk contravening the applicable regulations on their product packaging. Unfortunately, invalid health claims have appeared for products sold online, either in the product description or in reviews.

How can you determine whether a health claim is likely valid? Permitted claims are typically phrased judiciously. Examples are "Olive oil polyphenols contribute to the protection of blood lipids from oxidative stress" (permitted in the EU with certain restrictions) and "Adequate calcium and vitamin D throughout life, as part of a well-balanced diet, may reduce the risk of osteoporosis" (permitted in the US with certain restrictions). If you see a claim in unrestrained language indicating a complete cure for a serious disease, check it out by searching online.

Incidentally, apricot kernels not only don't cure cancer, as has been illegally claimed in the UK, but actually cause harm. Bitter kernels, including the powdered forms, should not be eaten because a substance in the kernels changes to cyanide after ingestion.

Warfarin and cod liver oil: medicines

If you are taking medicines, re-read the patient information leaflet to check for any interactions with food before making any major changes to your diet. Some foods and food supplements increase or decrease the effect of certain medicines. For example, cod liver oil interacts with the anticoagulant Warfarin.

Chapter 4: The lifelong gluten-free diet

If you have been diagnosed with a gluten-related disorder, your healthcare professional will have informed you that you need a lifelong gluten-free diet. Not a 10-day miracle diet. Not a fad diet. Not a diet backed by a commercial enterprise requiring you to buy a certain amount of their processed foods or supplements every month. Just a healthy, balanced diet that's also gluten-free. This chapter provides guidance on specific foods and food groups to include in the diet. It also covers what not to eat, when to eat, and how to eat.

What to eat

For each group of foods, we'll look at which foods within the group to eat, how often to eat them, and how to prepare or cook them.

It is important to get some foods from each group. Not all foods within each group are suitable for everyone, and personal biochemistry plays some part in this. Take Brussels sprouts — you either love them or hate them. If you're in the latter group, you probably have a certain variant of a gene that makes a chemical compound in Brussels sprouts taste bitter. Well, you don't have to eat Brussels sprouts if they are distasteful to you, but you do have to eat a variety of vegetables.

Vegetables

Eat at least three portions of vegetables every day, preferably more, including at least one green vegetable and one of another colour.

Vegetables provide fibre and vitamins. The leafy greens also provide calcium, magnesium, and non-heme iron. Vegetables are also a good source of potassium with little sodium, thus helping the potassium-to-sodium balance. Many vegetables also contain a lot of water and thus are good for hydration. They also encourage the growth of good bacteria in the gut.

Orange vegetables and leafy green vegetables contain fat-soluble vitamins (A, D, E, and K). To retain these vitamins, avoid frying sweet potato, carrots, broccoli, spinach, green cabbage, and kale. It's best to steam the leafy greens and boil the orange veg. Frying should be limited to light stir-frying.

Most other vegetables contain water-soluble vitamins (B and C), which are reduced when the foods containing them are cooked in water or exposed to heat or air for a long time. So most vegetables should be steamed, grilled, griddled, microwaved, stir fried, or roasted rather than boiled. If you do boil vegetables and are making a sauce or soup at the same time, reuse the water. Minimise the cooking time. Don't chop vegetables too finely, as that increases the surface area exposed to heat, air, and water.

But know your onions; in onions and their relatives garlic, leeks, and shallots, chopping releases a sulphur compound called allicin, which exhibits antimicrobial activity. Waiting ten minutes in between chopping and cooking helps to preserve the allicin. Include a moderate amount of vegetables from this family in your diet. In addition to the allicin, they provide a variety of vitamins and minerals and prebiotic fibre.

To retain all the vitamins in vegetables, eat them raw occasionally. Slices of celery, carrots, and bell peppers can be used as snacks. Many vegetables can be used raw in salads — not only lettuce, rocket (arugula), and cucumber but also carrots, green beans, cauliflower, red cabbage, chicory, parsnip, and some others. Some raw vegetables are more palatable if finely sliced or spiralized.

Tomatoes are a special case. Cooking actually increases the lycopene in them, though some of the vitamin C is lost. Or eat canned tomatoes, which are heated during the canning process. Yes, I know that tomatoes are technically fruits rather than vegetables, but I have grouped them with vegetables because most people use them as such. However, you might actually consider using them as a fruit — that is, try eating a few cherry tomatoes instead of another fruit when it's time for a fruity snack.

Potatoes are another special case. They are a good source of vitamin C and fibre, and they also provide other nutrients. They don't officially count toward your 5-a-day of vegetables and fruit because they are traditionally eaten as the carbohydrate part of a meal, like pasta or rice, rather than as a vegetable. However, some dietitians and nutritionists argue that they should count. Anyway, you can eat potatoes in moderation whether or not you count them. There are several points to note about the preparation of potatoes:

- To preserve the vitamin C in potatoes, bake rather than boil them.

- To benefit from the fibre in potatoes, eat the skins.

- To turn some of the digestible starch into the more beneficial resistant starch, chill boiled potatoes in the fridge overnight and eat them cold the next day. "Resistant" here means resisting digestion. Most starch is broken down into glucose during digestion, whereas resistant starch passes undigested from the small intestine to the large intestine, where it is fermented by gut bacteria. Thus, it acts like fibre.

- To avoid acrylamide, don't burn potatoes and limit your intake of potato crisps (which definitely don't count toward your 5-a-day). Acrylamide is a chemical that forms in potatoes when they are fried or baked at a temperature high enough to induce a reaction resulting in browning (the Maillard reaction). Acrylamide causes cancer in animals, which raises the concern that it might cause cancer in humans. Food regulators and the World Health Organization advise keeping exposure to acrylamide as low as reasonably practicable. They also encourage manufacturers to reduce the amount of acrylamide in processed foods. If you fry chips or heat oven chips at home, cook them to a light golden colour rather than browning them. (Certain other high-starch foods are also susceptible to acrylamide formation, in particular, wheat and rye during bread baking. But that's of no concern to those of us on a gluten-free diet.)

Frozen vegetables are fine. In fact, some vegetables taste better frozen than fresh because they are frozen within a few hours of picking, whereas fresh ones take several days to reach the supermarket shelf. Nonetheless, I make a point of getting fresh peas at least once a year just to have the satisfaction of popping them out of the pods.

Fruits

Eat fruit in moderation; one or two portions a day will suffice.

A portion may consist of small amounts of several different fruits.

The governments of many countries have run 5-a-day campaigns to encourage the consumption of fruit and vegetables. The advice is typically to eat five portions of fruit and/or vegetables every day. Many people have taken this to mean that any proportion of fruit and vegetables is fine, and they consume much more fruit than vegetables. Although fruit contains vitamins, minerals, and fibre, it also contains a lot of the sugar fructose. Therefore, large quantities of fruit are not good for you — especially if the fruit consumption is at the expense of vegetable consumption.

Fresh is best. Canned fruit is bad, due to the accompanying syrup. Dried fruits are bad because the sugar is concentrated and they may contain sulphites or be coated in palm oil or other undesirables. Also, it's easy to overeat them due to their small size. However, it's OK to have raisins or sultanas occasionally, perhaps mixed with nuts, because they have a good balance of minerals and vitamins and they confer several health benefits.

Whole is best. Fruit juices and smoothies are more sugary and less fibrous than fresh fruit because several pieces of fruit go into one glass of juice and the fibre gets left behind. Fruits are for eating, not drinking.

Dates may look like dried fruit but are nutritious fresh fruit — except the ones that are actually partially dried. Tell-tale signs are a glazed look and glucose syrup in the ingredients list, or the lack of a pit.

Bananas are good. They have many nutrients, including vitamins B6 and K, magnesium, and potassium. Unripe, greener bananas have a lot of resistant starch, whereas ripe bananas contain a lot of sugars (fructose, glucose, and sucrose); the starch is converted to sugars during ripening.

If you want to control weight or improve bowel health, unripe bananas are better. If you need a quick and convenient energy boost when halfway up a mountain or halfway round a golf course, a ripe banana is just the thing. To make full use of a banana, use the inside of the peel to clean leather shoes and bags.

Berries are good because they contain phytonutrients with antioxidant properties. They work at any time of the day: with muesli or porridge at breakfast, in a salad at lunchtime, or as a dessert after dinner.

Avocados are very good. The avocado is an unusual fruit in that it has very low sugar but around twenty vitamins and minerals, some phytonutrients, fibre, and monounsaturated fat. Many health benefits are claimed for avocados. Although definitive proof of some of these benefits is hard to find, such a nutrient-packed and tasty food must be good for you. Add sliced avocado to salads or gluten-free wraps or sandwiches. Spread it on rice cakes. Add mashed avocado to other ingredients to make a guacamole or an avocado mess of your own devising. Add half an avocado to a cooked breakfast instead of tomatoes.

Olives are fantastic, assuming you've reached the age at which you can acquire a taste for them, usually mid-20s. They have lots of anti-inflammatory polyphenols and flavonoids, along with monounsaturated fat. Green olives tend to have more polyphenols and more salt, whereas the riper black olives tend to have more oil. But they are otherwise similar in nutritional value and can be used interchangeably in recipes. Olives contain magnesium but that's gone in olive oil, so it's good to eat whole olives sometimes as well as using olive oil in marinades, dressings, and frying.

Although only a few fruits have been singled out for special attention here, they are all good in their own particular way. So do eat a variety of them, from the common or garden apple to the exotic papaya.

To get the maximum nutritional benefit from fruits, especially the vitamin C in citrus fruits, buy them as fresh as possible, consume them as soon as possible after purchase, and eat them raw — unless you have difficulty digesting fruits, in which case try stewing them. For fruits with edible peel, eat the peel too because that's where a lot of the goodness is stored — unless the fruit has been showcased on the street, where the peel absorbs pollution from passing traffic.

If you eat a fruit salad, serve it with cream because the fat in the cream reduces the rate at which the fruit sugars are released.

Legumes

Eat legumes occasionally if you like them and they like you and you have time for the long soaking required to improve their digestibility or are happy to eat them in the form of processed foods.

Legumes include beans, lentils, and chickpeas. They provide carbohydrates, minerals, and protein, though the protein is incomplete.

If you're gluten-free due to digestive disease or if eating legumes increases your intestinal gas to an uncomfortable level, limit your intake of legumes. But even people with delicate digestive systems may find that legumes can occasionally be put to good use: baked beans can substitute for tomatoes in a full English breakfast (go for a low-sugar, low-salt variety); hummus can be spread on a gluten-free cracker for lunch; and mangetout (snow peas or sugar snap peas) can add interest to a stir fry or can be steamed and served as a vegetable at dinner.

Meat

Eat meat on most days, especially on days when you are not having fish. During the course of a week, have both white and red meat.

Meat is the best source of complete protein and heme iron. It's also a very good source of zinc and B vitamins, including B12. These are all critical for physical and mental health.

Some people worry that eating red meat may be bad for their health, but the trick is to control the three P's: portion size, processing, and preparation.

- Portion size. Examples of healthy portion sizes are three thin slices of roasted meat, half a beef steak, and a patty-sized (rather than burger-sized) cake of minced beef.

- Processing. Limit your intake of processed meat, to avoid nitrates and nitrites.

- Preparation. Don't chargrill or barbecue meat, to avoid the formation of harmful chemicals.

Get the best quality meat you can afford. It may be difficult to find out how animals have been reared and how much of the meat consists of water. But there's a rule of thumb you can use to assess meat quality: each meat should have a distinctive flavour. If someone blindfolds you and feeds you, say, a cube of pork and a cube of chicken and you can't tell the difference, something is wrong. If you find that a cut of meat is bland when eaten on its own and must be drowned in a tangy sauce in order to be appetizing, something is wrong.

Fish and shellfish

Eat fish two or three times per week, including oily fish at least twice per week.

All fish and shellfish contain a good quantity of protein (though not the complete protein found in meat), along with other nutrients. The oily fish additionally contain vitamin D and Omega-3 oil. Common oily fish in Europe are mackerel, salmon, tuna, sardines, trout, and herring. When tuna is canned, the Omega-3 is severely reduced, so go for a fresh tuna steak. However, the other oily fish are OK canned.

Oily fish contain fat-soluble vitamins. To retain these vitamins, bake, grill, or poach; don't fry.

White fish contain more water-soluble vitamins. To retain these vitamins, bake, fry, or microwave; don't poach.

Or have raw fish in sushi, if good gluten-free sushi is available in your neighbourhood.

Some people worry that fish may be contaminated with mercury, but the selenium in fish goes some way to counteracting the effect of mercury (and scientists have found that fish seem to accumulate more selenium from their environment if exposed to mercury). The consensus seems to be that the benefits of eating fish two or three times a week outweigh the risks.

Another concern is the sustainability of fishing. Seafood products with the international Marine Stewardship Council ecolabel ("Certified sustainable seafood MSC") should be fished in accordance with principles of sustainability. However, some environmental organizations and scientists believe that this is a weak certification. So, if you are really interested in sustainability, look for information on the particular fisheries where your fish comes from.

Cereals and pseudo-cereals

Use quinoa, rice, and buckwheat as staple foods, eating at least one of them almost every day and all of them during the course of the week. Include quinoa at least three times a week. (The reason for the selection of this trio of staples is in the "Replacing the work of wheat" section.) Eat gluten-free oats as often as you want, if you can tolerate oats. You can also eat other uncontaminated non-gluten-containing cereals and pseudo-cereals. (Exclude wheat, rye, and barley, which do contain gluten.)

Rice grains and quinoa grains should be rinsed through a sieve before use. Buckwheat groats should be soaked in water for six hours or overnight and then rinsed before use. Flours ground from these three foods can be used in the same way as any other flour.

Cooking quinoa is simple. For 4 portions, boil 1 cup of quinoa in 2 cups of water for 15 minutes or until all the water has been absorbed. You can keep cooked quinoa for up to 5 days. Let it cool and then store in an airtight container in the fridge. Buying quinoa should not be difficult because it is grown in South America, North America, Europe, Africa, and Asia.

Buying buckwheat can be difficult. In the UK, many bags of buckwheat flour carry warnings that they contain, or may contain, gluten. To me, the mere existence of such products is perplexing. Buckwheat is not part of traditional UK cuisine; in all my pre-gluten-free years, I never once encountered a recipe that called for buckwheat and never saw buckwheat flour in the shops. It was only when I became gluten-free that I looked for it in specialist shops and online. So I imagine that a large part of the UK market for buckwheat consists of people on a gluten-free diet. Yet we cannot have the contaminated stuff. So who is that stuff for? Fortunately, you can get gluten-free buckwheat online.

There was controversy for years over whether it is safe for celiacs to eat oats because studies gave conflicting results. Oats do not contain gluten, but they do contain a similar protein called avenin. In 2007, a systematic review of earlier studies on oats and celiac disease concluded that most celiacs can beneficially include oats in their diet, though a small percentage of celiacs may be sensitive to oats.[24] The authors of the review say that conflicting results from earlier studies may have been partly due to contamination of oats with wheat; most oats become contaminated with gluten from other grains during harvesting or milling. More recent research also concluded that pure oats (those labelled "gluten-free") are safe for most celiacs. As a result, both Health Canada and the UK's National Institute for Health and Care Excellence (NICE) revised their guidance in 2015 and now say that it's OK for celiacs to eat oats. Furthermore, there is no longer any suggestion that there is a daily limit on consumption or that you have to be gluten-free for some months before reintroducing oats.

Eat only oats explicitly labelled as gluten-free. These are kept away from gluten-containing grains during growing and processing and are tested for gluten. If something bad happens every time you eat gluten-free oats, try switching to a different brand because different oat cultivars have different properties. If bad things still happen, check with your doctor whether you have to avoid oats.

If you can tolerate oats, it is beneficial to include them in your diet because they are very nutritious. Oats contain several B vitamins, and several minerals, including magnesium, iron, and zinc. They also contain beta-glucan, which is a type of soluble fibre that contributes to the maintenance of normal blood cholesterol levels and digestive health. Consumption of a substantial amount of beta-glucan from oats as part of a meal contributes to the reduction of the blood glucose rise after that meal. If you previously ate wheat breakfast cereals and are looking for an alternative source of nutrients at the breakfast table, oat is your friend. In fact, you can have much tastier breakfasts with oats then you ever had with processed wheat cereals; you can use them to make porridge in winter and muesli in summer. You can also use oats in some cake recipes.

Eggs

Eat at least three eggs per week. Even better, eat one or two almost every day.

Eggs are good for you. Earlier advice to limit egg consumption was withdrawn because our understanding of cholesterol has changed and eggs have changed. A nutrient analysis conducted in the UK in 2012 showed that chicken eggs in 2011 contained more vitamin D and selenium than in the late 1980s and slightly less fat, due to changes in chicken feed and egg production methods.[25] The report also confirms the other nutrients in eggs, including protein, fat (all types), vitamin A, various B vitamins, vitamin E, folate, various minerals including iodine, zinc, calcium, and magnesium, and some phytonutrients.

British eggs are not only more nutritious now but also safer because chickens are now vaccinated against salmonella.

There are lots of things you can do with eggs: boil, scramble, poach, fry, make into an omelette or frittata, drop into an egg-shaped hole in a vegetable bake, serve with ham and chips, use in cake recipes, use hard boiled and quartered in a kedgeree or in a salade niçoise, go to work on one. If you want Scotch eggs, however, you have to make them yourself with sausage meat extracted from gluten-free sausages and rice crumbs.

Duck eggs can be useful if you want a change from chicken eggs or if you are allergic to chicken eggs but not duck eggs. (If you have a severe allergy, first check with your doctor whether it is appropriate for you to try other eggs.) Duck eggs contain similar nutrients to chicken eggs in greater quantities. This is partly due to their larger size and partly due to having more nutrients per gram. They can be used in the same ways as chicken eggs, except for making meringues; the egg white doesn't stiffen well enough when beaten.

Incidentally, some chicken eggs in some parts of the world are marketed as containing Omega-3, due to the use of chicken feed containing Omega-3. However, the type and quantity of Omega-3 is usually unspecified. It may be largely in the ALA form, and the amount of any DHA may be too low to make a significant contribution to the diet. So stick to oily fish for Omega-3.

Dairy products

Eat two or three portions of dairy products every day. Include live yogurt at least three times per week.

Examples of dairy product portions are a 200 ml glass of milk, a single-portion pot of yogurt, and a matchbox-sized piece of cheese.

3-a-day dairy campaigns have been run in several countries, with the aim of reducing the incidence of calcium deficiency and other nutritional deficiencies. In some countries, including Ireland, 3-a-day dairy advice has been incorporated into official nutritional guidelines. Regrettably, the UK is an exception. In December 2015, the UK Dairy All-Party Parliamentary Group wrote to the Department of Health to ask for the implementation of a 3-a-day programme, as part of an enquiry for a report. It has to be said that one aim of the APPG is to support the UK dairy industry, but the report nonetheless makes good nutritional points about the consumption of dairy products.[26] In a single week in March 2016, the APPG published its report and a Department of Health agency, Public Health England, published revised nutritional guidance (the "Eatwell Guide") in which it actually reduced the recommended intake of dairy products.

Anyway, having three portions a day of milk and/or yogurt and/or cheese is the best way to get the recommended intake of calcium. These foods also provide protein and a variety of vitamins and minerals. Live yogurt additionally provides good bacteria. Butter and cream can also be included in the diet, though they have a different nutritional profile; they contain more fat, less calcium, and less lactose than cheese and milk.

When buying milk, you must decide on the type — low fat, middling fat, whole milk, or unhomogenized (cream floats to the top) whole milk. The received wisdom in the late 20th century was that low-fat varieties are healthier. Not only is fat in general no longer considered bad but also the particular types of saturated fatty acids in milk are actually claimed to confer health benefits, particularly regarding the risk of cardiovascular disease. Also note that when fat is removed from milk, some of the vitamin A goes with it. It's up to you. If you're buying milk for use in a milk pudding or any recipe requiring milk, whole milk gives better results. If you're buying it for drinking on its own or adding to hot beverages or breakfast cereals, go with your personal preference.

When buying cheese, check the salt content because some cheeses are very salty. If this applies to your preferred type of cheese, it's usually possible to find a different brand of the same type with less salt.

When buying yogurt, choose natural yogurt with live bacteria and change brands occasionally. The ingredients list should contain only milk and live cultures (for example, bifidobacterium and lactobacillus acidophilus). If there's anything else — sugar, glucose syrup, fructose, fruit, tapioca starch, maize starch, cream, gums, acidity regulators, stabilizers, flavourings, sweeteners — it's not proper yogurt. It's dessert. Try to re-educate your palate to accept the sour taste of natural yogurt. If you insist on a sweet taste, get a natural yogurt and serve it with fresh fruit. Or make a fruit lassi. Changing brands occasionally increases the chance that you will get different strains of bacteria and that a proportion of them will exit your stomach alive and set up home in your gut. Even if you doubt that yogurt improves your gut bacteria, eat it anyway because it provides calcium and protein and may serve as a comfort food.

Goat's or sheep's milk/yogurt/cheese/butter provide similar nutrition to the equivalent products from cows. They can be useful if you want to add variety to the diet or if you are allergic to cow's milk but not goat's or sheep's milk. (This refers to an allergy to milk proteins, *not* to lactose intolerance. If you have a severe cow's milk allergy, first check with your doctor whether it is appropriate for you to try other milks.)

Nuts and seeds

Eat a handful of nuts and/or seeds, or the equivalent in nut/seed butter, several days a week.

Nuts and seeds provide protein, saturated fat, and various vitamins and minerals. One of their functions in the gluten-free diet is replacing the magnesium that "normal" people get from wheat. Many fruits and vegetables contain magnesium but not at the levels found in nuts and seeds. Also, some magnesium is lost during the cooking of vegetables. So you definitely need to include nuts and seeds in your diet.

Although some nutrients are common to most nuts and seeds, others make a star appearance in some nuts and seeds but only a minor appearance in others and a no-show in the rest. Therefore, it's important to eat a variety of nuts and seeds during the course of a week. Some options are walnuts, macadamia nuts, almonds, hazelnuts, pecans, Brazil nuts, pine nuts, pumpkin seeds, and sesame seeds.

There are many ways to enjoy nuts and seeds. You can have them as a snack. You can sprinkle them on a salad. Pine nuts or cashew nuts can be added to a stir fry in the last minute or two. Lightly crushed walnuts can be baked into cakes. Nut butters can be spread on gluten-free bread or rice crackers or included in a Pad Thai (where almond butter can replace the peanuts if you don't eat peanuts).

But what if you find nuts difficult to digest? Nuts contain phytic acid, which binds to iron, calcium, zinc and other minerals during digestion, thus reducing the bioavailability of the minerals. Nuts also contain digestive enzyme inhibitors, making indigestion a possibility. To prevent this, either limit your intake to just a handful of nuts on just a few days a week or soak them first. Soaking reduces the phytic acid. It also softens nuts, which is good if you want to include them in your diet but have weak teeth.

To soak nuts, cover them with warm water and add salt — a tablespoon of salt per four cups of nuts. Leave to soak for seven hours or overnight and then drain off and discard the water and rinse the nuts through a strainer with fresh cold water. If you're using the nuts immediately, you're done. If you're using them within 24 hours, dry them with a clean towel or kitchen paper and refrigerate them. If you plan to use them over the next couple of weeks, thoroughly dehydrate them before refrigerating because wet nuts go mouldy. To dehydrate soaked nuts, put them on a baking sheet in the oven on a very low temperature (about 50° C / 122° F) for 12 hours.

Although nuts and seeds can be expensive, a serving is only a handful. And you can reduce the cost by buying large bags of several different types of nuts and seeds and making up your own mixture as required.

Oils and fats

Keep a supply of olive oil, sesame oil, and a solid fat or coconut oil at home ready for use in food preparation and cooking, along with your preferred choice of other healthy oils and fats.

If you always have bottles of olive oil and sesame oil at home, you will be ready for most dishes requiring oil. Both can be used in marinades and for frying. Olive oil can also be used in salad dressings and drizzled over vegetables. Sesame oil can be used in Asian dishes and drizzled over hummus or other dips to add a pleasing, nutty, toasty tang.

Rapeseed oil (canola oil) can be used in everyday cooking in which no special flavour is required.

Nut and seed oils, such as walnut oil and flaxseed oil, are also healthy and tasty but more expensive and with a shorter shelf life and not suitable for cooking. For a special treat, buy a small bottle and keep it in the fridge. To get best value from it before it goes rancid, tip it liberally into dressings until it's used up.

Because oxidation can occur if oils are exposed to light or air, put the top on the bottle and return it to the cupboard immediately after use. Dark bottles are better than clear ones, in terms of minimizing exposure to light (including before purchase). Do not reuse oils, as re-heating causes further chemical breakdown. When frying with oil, keep the temperature below the oil's smoking point.

The best fats for frying and roasting, in terms of producing the least amount of harmful chemicals when heated, are the solid fats — butter, lard (pork fat), goose fat, duck fat — and coconut oil. So always have at least one of these in the fridge (or in the cupboard, in the case of coconut oil).

Of course, some fatty cuts of meat can be cooked largely in their own juices.

Chocolate

Eat two or three squares of dark chocolate with a high percentage of cocoa solids, or a teaspoon of unsweetened cocoa powder in hot chocolate, on most days.

When I say "chocolate", I mean something that meets the definition of chocolate that was proposed by the EU in 2000 but shamefully vetoed by the UK — that is, something in which the only fat is cocoa butter. I also mean something in which the only other ingredients are cocoa solids, a small amount of sugar, and an emulsifier. The percentage of cocoa solids must be high (60% or more) because it's the cocoa solids that contain the beneficial flavonoids, namely, catechins.

Here are links to a selection of news items reporting on the health benefits of eating dark chocolate. You may like to follow them and see if you can spot a pattern. (The answer follows the list.)

- *Chocolate helps blood vessels*
  (http://news.bbc.co.uk/1/hi/health/3756997.stm, 1 Jun 2004)
- *Chocolate may cut heart disease*
  (http://news.bbc.co.uk/1/hi/health/4535974.stm, 20 Dec 2005)
- *Chocolate cuts blood clot risk*
  (http://news.bbc.co.uk/1/hi/health/6146070.stm, 15 Nov 2006)
- *Chocolate can cut blood pressure and help heart*
  (http://news.bbc.co.uk/1/hi/health/8593887.stm, 30 Mar 2010)
- *Dark chocolate can be good for the heart*
  (http://www.bbc.co.uk/news/health-10986625, 16 Aug 2010)

- *Chocolate may protect the brain and heart*
  (http://www.bbc.co.uk/news/health-14679497, 30 Aug 2011)
- *Dark chocolate may lower blood pressure*
  (http://www.bbc.co.uk/news/health-19241924, 15 Aug 2012)

The pattern is that, whenever a study finds a benefit from eating chocolate, a spokesperson for the British Heart Foundation says you shouldn't eat it. It's essentially the same reaction every time and it's focused on sugar, calories, and saturated fat.

Regarding sugar, the British Heart Foundation says that chocolate contains too much sugar. I say that dark chocolate doesn't contain as much sugar as milk chocolate or white chocolate. And most of the studies used dark chocolate.

Regarding calories, the British Heart Foundation says that chocolate contains too many calories. I say that calories represent energy and recovering celiacs need energy. It's true that you should go easy on the calories if you have already reached a normal weight, especially if you aren't physically active. But the studies show that you only need a few squares of chocolate per day to gain the cardiovascular benefits. The BHF's reaction would be appropriate if the researchers were recommending that you binge on chocolate, but they aren't.

Regarding saturated fat, well, at the time the British Heart Foundation commented on the stories, its spokespersons obviously subscribed to the contemporary belief that saturated fat is bad for you. Subsequently, the BHF co-funded some research about fat consumption and heart disease — but they wanted to repudiate it when it didn't give the results they had expected. That story is reported here:

- *Should I avoid saturated fat?* (http://www.bbc.co.uk/news/health-26622399, 17 Mar 2014)

The story says that the analysis of dozens of studies did not yield clear evidence that switching from saturated fats to monounsaturated and polyunsaturated fats reduced the risk of cardiovascular disease. The BHF was surprised and wants to see more research before changing its dietary advice. Anyway, saturated fat isn't particularly relevant here because dark chocolate has a high amount of non-fat cocoa solids.

The BHF recommends eating fruits and vegetables instead of chocolate on the basis that they also contain flavonoids. Although fruits and vegetables should be part of your diet for other reasons, they cannot substitute for chocolate because they contain different flavonoids. Only a few fruits and berries contain catechins and then in much lower quantities than in chocolate — though you could substitute green tea if you prefer because it contains a good supply of catechins.

Let's wait and see when the BHF's dietary advice changes. Meanwhile, don't get me started on their track record on animal testing.

But surely chocolate is bad for your teeth? Although chocolate bars contain sugar, they are not as bad for your teeth as confectionery because cocoa butter coats the teeth, protecting them from acids that cause tooth decay. Another ingredient of chocolate, theobromine, helps to remineralize teeth and there are toothpastes coming on to the market containing compounds in which one ingredient is derived from theobromine. No dentist will actually encourage you to eat chocolate. But, if you are going to have something sweet, chocolate is preferable to confectionery. You can verify this yourself. One day, have a small bar of chocolate (just chocolate, as defined above) and check how your teeth feel an hour or two later. The next day, have some confectionery (such as fruit gums or nougat) and check how your teeth feel an hour or two later. Even though chocolate is not as harmful for the teeth as confectionery, you will ideally eat your chocolate ration immediately after dinner and then clean your teeth.

Avoid milk chocolate. Given that dark chocolate typically contains 75–85% cocoa solids and milk chocolate typically contains only 25–30% cocoa solids, what do you suppose makes up the difference? If you think it's mostly milk, or even milk powder, think again. It's mostly sugar. Check the label; you will likely find "sugar" at the top of the ingredients list and "sugars" at over 50 g per 100 g in the nutrition declaration. Unlike dark chocolate, milk chocolate is not a health food.

Homemade hot chocolate with fresh milk is another matter. You can make great hot chocolate by simply putting a teaspoon of cocoa powder and a cup of milk into a saucepan, *without* adding sugar, and heating it to just below boiling point, stirring continuously. Now you've got a good part of your calcium ration from fresh milk instead of powdered milk and no refined sugar. For a good night's sleep, drink it after dinner. For an even better night's sleep, stir in some mashed banana after pouring it into a mug. The soporific effect is probably due to all three ingredients containing tryptophan, which raises the level of serotonin, which produces melatonin, which regulates the daily sleep-wake cycle.

Ideally, cocoa powder should be non-Dutched, though it's nearly always Dutched. The Dutching process makes cocoa powder more alkaline, usually by adding potassium carbonate. This process makes the powder taste less bitter but substantially reduces the amount of polyphenols, thus diminishing the health benefits.

Does chocolate have any other benefits? As an intelligent person, you may be wondering whether eating chocolate will help you to win a Nobel Prize. If so, see "Does chocolate make you clever?" here: http://www.bbc.co.uk/news/magazine-20356613. Admittedly, the article is about spurious correlation but it's enjoyable.

By the way, the UK's veto of the EU chocolate legislation was aimed at protecting British manufacturers of inferior chocolate, but it didn't help in the long term. In 2010, Cadbury was bought by the American company Kraft Foods, which promised pre-takeover that it would retain factories in the UK but promptly moved production elsewhere, making UK staff redundant. Kraft Foods subsequently split into two companies, with the Cadbury brand going to Mondelez International. Mondelez then annoyed British customers and taxpayers by changing the recipes of the products and avoiding UK tax. If the proposed EU legislation had been approved, Cadbury and other British chocolate manufacturers would have had a decade of upping their game and might not have been such an attractive takeover target for manufacturers of down-market foods.

Having recommended a daily chocolate ration, I have to report that finding gluten-free chocolate in the UK is difficult. Most of the brands commonly available in supermarkets and corner shops contain or may contain gluten and/or aren't proper chocolate. Even some up-market brands contain gluten.

You may find something labelled as gluten-free chocolate in the Free From section at a supermarket. But check whether it is actually chocolate. Just look at the ingredients list of a UK supermarket's own brand of "Freefrom" chocolate:

> "Sugar, Cocoa Butter, Cocoa Mass, Rice Syrup, Inulin, Coconut Oil, Rice Flour, Flavourings, Emulsifier: **Soya** Lecithin."

Why, oh why, would anyone put rice flour in a chocolate bar? Rice flour is legitimately used in some Free From products, for the purpose of replacing wheat flour — in cakes, for example. But normal chocolate bars don't have wheat flour as an intentional ingredient, so there's nothing to replace. And what's with the inulin, coconut oil, and flavourings? If a chocolate bar is made from good quality cocoa mass and cocoa butter, it doesn't need any of these extras. Why can't they simply make a chocolate bar with the normal ingredients but without gluten contamination?

Herbs and spices

Use fresh or dried culinary herbs and spices in moderation to bring out the flavour of some foods.

Note that many herbs are medicines, not foods. Indeed, the active substances in some pharmaceutical medicines are synthetic versions of the active substances in some herbs. If you use medicinal herbs in food preparation, you might be medicating yourself rather than feeding yourself — and you cannot be sure how much of the active substance you are getting because that depends on the growing conditions. So stick to the traditional culinary herbs such as parsley, sage, rosemary, and thyme.

You can also make your own herbal teas by simply steeping fresh herbs or spices in hot water. Some refreshing options are a few mint leaves, a sprig of parsley, or some chopped or grated ginger root.

Anecdotally, fresh ginger tea is said to be good for calming the digestive system after getting glutened.

Salt

Aim for a moderate salt intake of 2–3 g per day, up to a maximum of 6 g. (6 g is about one teaspoon.)

This judgement of a "moderate intake" strikes a balance among official dietary recommendations from various countries and recommendations from other sources.

You can moderate your salt intake by avoiding processed foods and checking the labels on any processed foods you do have. If you eat a highly salted meal or snack on a given day, don't add salt in cooking or at the table for other meals on that day. If you eat only fresh foods, add some salt in cooking or at the table.

A high salt intake can lead to high blood pressure, but a very low salt intake can also cause health problems. Sodium is needed for nerve transmission and muscle contraction, chloride is needed for making hydrochloric acid in the stomach, and both are needed for fluid balance. So do moderate your salt intake but don't try to eliminate it altogether.

Note that sea salt is still salt, even if the marketing messages imply that it's healthier than regular table salt. Some unprocessed sea salts do contain extra minerals — those naturally present in the salt on the coast from which it is gathered. But given that most of the minerals will be present only in trace amounts and you will consume only a small amount of the salt daily, it's unlikely that switching to unprocessed sea salt will make a significant difference to your health.

If you think a meal would be too bland with only a moderate amount of salt, season it with herbs or lemon or lime. Also, use the most flavoursome food you can afford when preparing meals. Then each ingredient will deliver its own distinctive tang.

Vinegar

Use vinegar in cooking or in dressings as desired, being sure to choose a gluten-free one: cider vinegar, wine vinegar, balsamic vinegar, or rice vinegar.

Avoid malt vinegar because it's made from malted barley that has *not* been distilled and thus not had the gluten removed. (Some people say that most or all of the gluten is removed during other parts of the vinegar-making process, such as fermentation, and that the final product is safe for celiacs. Then again, some assays used to test for the presence of gluten are not very sensitive to barley gluten. So malt vinegar is best avoided.)

Moving on to distilled white vinegar — well, it depends on what it has been distilled from. If it has been distilled from corn or potato, it will be gluten-free. If it has been distilled from a gluten-containing grain, it depends on how much of the gluten is removed by the distillation process. Check the label.

If you're tempted by flavoured vinegars (tarragon vinegar, raspberry vinegar, etc.), check the label in case part of the flavouring comes from wheat.

There's a complication with rice vinegar. The pale-coloured rice vinegar on sale in supermarkets is gluten-free. But be aware that the rice vinegar concoction used in Japanese cuisine and in some other Asian cuisines often contains barley or wheat too. This is sometimes called black rice vinegar.

If "vinegar" is in the ingredients list for another type of food product, it is usually cider vinegar and thus safe. But if the ingredients list says "malt vinegar (from barley)", avoid it.

Fermented food

Eat a forkful of a fermented food once a day at the start of your main meal.

A forkful of sauerkraut or kimchi at the start of a meal could help to improve digestion and general health because these fermented foods contain both probiotics and prebiotics. Choose non-pasteurized varieties because pasteurization destroys the good bacteria. Fermented foods have to contain salt but some contain more than necessary, so do check the salt content.

To avoid digestive discomfort from excessive fermentation, don't overdose on prebiotics. Do not, for example, eat a lot of sauerkraut and drink kefir and take a probiotic supplement.

Honey and syrups

If you eat honey or syrups, do so sparingly.

Honey consists mainly of fructose and glucose, agave nectar is very high in fructose, and neither offer any significant amount of any vitamins or minerals. Maple syrup is high in sucrose, though it also contains zinc, magnesium, calcium, and some B vitamins. Consequently, these sweeteners should be reserved for occasional treats.

Water

Start the day with a mug of cold tap water and drink more water during the day. Taper off to sips of water during the evening.

The body is about 60% water, which must be regularly replenished. However, the widespread advice to drink a specific volume of water per day is not backed by scientific evidence. The requirement for water varies from person to person and from day to day. Factors affecting your personal requirement include the temperature and humidity where you hang out, the water and salt in your food, and how much you exercise and sweat.

If you feel thirsty, you need to drink more. Even if your sense of thirst is not reliable — it can diminish with age or as a result of habitually ignoring it — you can still ascertain whether you are drinking enough: if you are properly hydrated, the urine is pale yellow. If it's dark, you need to drink more. Otherwise, you are at greater risk of urinary tract infections, constipation, and kidney stones. If it's bright yellow, you took a vitamin supplement containing more B vitamins than you need.

In some places, the tap water provides 10–20% of your daily requirement for magnesium — if you live in a hard water area and the balance of magnesium and calcium in the water is good and you drink plenty of it and you cook with it and you don't have a water softener and you don't use a water filter. Check your water company's website for details of the water composition in your area. UK residents, note that the calcium-to-magnesium ratio in the hard water areas is typically much greater than 2:1, so the water won't help your magnesium status.

In most parts of the developed world, tap water is better for your health than bottled water because (1) many bottled waters contain worse sodium-to-potassium and calcium-to-magnesium ratios than tap water, (2) tap water is more stringently regulated regarding testing for bacterial contamination, and (3) substances can leach from plastic bottles into the water. Especially avoid flavoured bottled waters, which contain artificial flavourings and either sugar or artificial sweeteners.

Bottled water is not only bad for your health but also bad for the environment because (1) millions of barrels of crude oil are used every year to make the plastic bottles, (2) many of these bottles end up in landfill sites or oceans, where they take many years to decompose, and (3) many resources are used in transporting bottled water around the world.

If you need to carry water around with you, it's best to buy a stainless steel bottle and fill it from the tap.

If you insist on having branded water, have Volvic. Of the brands widely available in the UK and France, Volvic has the healthiest balance of minerals. It's also available in other countries. To find the mineral content of bottled waters available in other parts of the world, use the Fine Waters site (www.finewaters.com).

Tea and coffee

If you drink tea or coffee, have no more than three cups per day.

Both tea and coffee are generally considered beneficial in moderation but harmful in excess for various reasons.

"Tea" here means actual tea from the *camellia sinensis* plant. Note that tea contains more caffeine than you think.

Summary of what to eat

Eat at least three portions of **vegetables** *every day, preferably more, including at least one green vegetable and one of another colour.*

Eat **fruit** *in moderation; one or two portions a day will suffice.*

Eat **legumes** *occasionally.*

Eat **meat** *on most days, especially on days when you are not having fish. During the course of a week, have both white and red meat.*

Eat **fish** *two or three times per week, including oily fish at least twice per week.*

Use **quinoa, rice, and buckwheat** *as staple foods, eating at least one of them almost every day and all of them during the course of the week. Include quinoa at least three times a week. Eat* **gluten-free oats** *as often as you want, if you can tolerate oats. You can also eat* **other uncontaminated non-gluten-containing cereals and pseudo-cereals.** *(Exclude wheat, rye, and barley, which do contain gluten,)*

Eat at least three **eggs** *per week. Even better, eat one or two almost every day.*

Eat two or three portions of **dairy products** *every day. Include live yogurt at least three times per week.*

Eat a handful of **nuts and/or seeds,** *or the equivalent in nut/seed butter, several days a week.*

Keep a supply of olive oil, sesame oil, and a solid fat or coconut oil at home ready for use in food preparation and cooking, along with your preferred choice of other healthy **oils and fats.**

Eat two or three squares of **dark chocolate** *with a high percentage of cocoa solids, or a teaspoon of unsweetened cocoa powder in hot chocolate, on most days.*

Use fresh or dried culinary **herbs and spices** *in moderation to bring out the flavour of some foods.*

Aim for a moderate **salt** *intake of 2–3 g per day, up to a maximum of 6 g. (6 g is about one teaspoon.)*

Use **vinegar** *in cooking or in dressings as desired, being sure to choose a gluten-free one.*

Eat a forkful of a **fermented food** *once a day at the start of your main meal.*

If you eat **honey or syrups**, *do so sparingly.*

Start the day with a mug of cold tap **water** *and drink more water during the day. Taper off to sips of water during the evening.*

If you drink **tea or coffee**, *have no more than three cups per day.*

What not to eat

Certain foods are best avoided not because they contain gluten but because they have little or no place in any healthy diet.

Processed food

If you think this section doesn't apply to you because you already avoid processed food, why do you read food labels? Fresh food isn't labelled. Is it possible that you eat more processed food than you think? Is there a cupboard in your kitchen full of cans and packets rather than cups and plates? Is there a shelf in your fridge full of jars rather than dairy products and salad vegetables? Do you sometimes prepare a meal of fresh meat and vegetables and then serve it with chutney or ketchup? The chutney or ketchup is in a bottle. The contents of the bottle are processed in a factory in between being picked from the field or orchard and being poured over your dinner.

Most people accept that fresh vegetables are better than canned vegetables and fresh fruit is better than dried fruit and a meal prepared from fresh ingredients is better than a ready meal. But when it comes to butter vs. yellow spreads or a freshly cooked breakfast vs. a breakfast cereal, some people believe the processed option to be healthier. Personally, I believe that choosing fresh food over processed food is the best choice every time. And now many nutrition experts say that butter is better for you than margarine or other yellow spreads and that breakfast cereals have too much salt and sugar and not enough goodness.

The deciding factor for me is that margarine and breakfast cereals simply don't taste like food. If you think they do taste good, that's due to the power of conditioning. If you've been eating cereal for breakfast every day for years, try eating fresh food for breakfast for a month and then try the cereal again and see what you think.

Another problem with processed food is that you cannot be sure exactly what you are eating, as has been demonstrated by various food scandals. A food manufacturer may buy raw ingredients in good faith and label the resultant products accordingly, only to find that someone in the supply chain adulterated the ingredients. A prime example is the European horsemeat scandal of 2013, in which beef burgers and other beef products were found to contain horsemeat. There were issues of deception and food safety; people who prefer not to eat horsemeat were deceived into eating it, and a veterinary drug that is dangerous to humans may have been given to horses that were not intended as food-producing animals but that ended up in the food chain.

Lightly processed foods can be as problematic as heavily processed ones. For example, herbs and spices contaminated with nut proteins (especially cumin contaminated with peanut protein and paprika contaminated with almond protein) turned up in various European countries in early 2015, posing a health risk for people with nut allergies. In the UK, contaminated spices then made their way into supermarket own brand ready meals, resulting in product recalls due to the undeclared presence of allergens. One UK supermarket had to recall its Blackened Salmon Portions. Now, blackened salmon is basically fresh food, right? I mean, it's just salmon that has been brushed with oil or butter and coated with a spice mix. But this particular incarnation (or should that be impescation?) had to be recalled because the paprika used in its manufacture was contaminated with almond protein. If you don't have a nut allergy, you may not be concerned about this particular scandal. But in case a future food scandal involves gluten contamination, it's best to buy truly fresh food and season it yourself.

Even if the ingredients are exactly as listed, gluten-free processed food is usually worse than normal processed food. I'm going to take you on a journey starting at a traditional recipe for a fresh Bakewell Tart, calling in at a "normal" processed tart, and finishing at a gluten-free processed tart.

Here are the ingredients of a traditional, fresh Bakewell Tart.

Shortcrust pastry (wheat flour, butter, water), raspberry jam, butter, sugar, ground almonds, flaked almonds, eggs, almond extract, icing sugar (optional, for dusting).

Here are the ingredients of a UK supermarket's own-brand boxed set of Bakewell Tarts, as at June 2015.

"Fortified wheat flour (**wheat** flour, calcium carbonate, iron, niacin, thiamin), unsalted butter (**milk**), sugar, raspberry jam (14%) (maize glucose-fructose syrup, raspberries, gelling agent pectin, acidity regulators citric acid and sodium citrates), pasteurised free range **egg**, ground **almonds**, maize flour, **almonds**, wheat glucose-fructose syrup, raising agents diphosphates and sodium carbonate, flavouring, salt, acidity regulators calcium chloride, citric acid and sodium citrates, gelling agent pectin."

Here are the ingredients of the same supermarket's own-brand boxed set of Gluten-Free Cherry Bakewells at the same time. (A Cherry Bakewell Tart is topped with a thin layer of soft icing and one cherry but . should otherwise be the same.)

"Sugar, palm oil, rice flour, water, strawberry jam (8%) (corn glucose syrup, sucrose syrup, strawberry puree, humectant vegetable glycerine, acidity regulators citric acid and trisodium citrate, gelling agent pectin, flavourings, colour anthocyanins), potato starch, maize starch, glace cherry (4%) (sugar, cherry, corn glucose fructose syrup, colour anthocyanins, acidity regulator citric acid, preservative **sulphur dioxide**), rapeseed oil, dextrose monohydrate, corn glucose syrup, maize flour, preservative potassium sorbate, emulsifiers sorbitan monostearate, sunflower lecithin, mono- and diglycerides of fatty acids and polyglycerol esters of fatty acids, flavouring, humectant vegetable glycerine, free range whole **egg**, ground **almonds**, acetic acid, gelling agent pectin, raising agents calcium phosphates, potassium carbonate and potassium phosphates, beet sugar fibre, dried free range **egg**, stabilisers xanthan gum and hydroxypropyl methyl cellulose, stearic acid, salt, acidity regulator potassium hydroxide."

I rest my case.

Additives

"We are living in a world today where lemonade is made from artificial flavors and furniture polish is made from real lemons." – Alfred Newman.

If you do eat processed food, it is generally best to choose products with few additives. Although all allowed food additives are assessed for safety, it is sometimes necessary to do reassessments. Moreover, good food doesn't need much in the way of chemical boosts.

Some additives are needed for good reasons such as preservation. And some are nutritious. For example, in the international numbering scheme for additives, 300 is ascorbic acid, which is vitamin C; 101 is riboflavin, which is vitamin B2; and 163 is anthocyanin, which is a phytonutrient.

(These are the numbers that are prefixed with "E" on food labels in the EU and presented unadorned on labels in Australia and New Zealand and not used at all in North America because Americans and Canadians like to do things their own way. A simple list of the numbers and functions of these additives is available at www.food.gov.uk/science/additives/enumberlist.)

Trans fats

Trans fats turn up when liquid oils are processed into a solid form for use in spreads and some other processed foods and fast food. They have an unusual chemical structure compared to other unsaturated fats, and consumption of them is associated with increased risk of coronary heart disease.

Although small amounts of trans fats occur naturally in some foods, the main concern is with industrially produced trans fats because they are consumed in larger amounts by some sub-groups of the population.

Some countries have banned industrially produced trans fats. In the US, the FDA introduced a ban in 2018. In 2019, the EU set a limit of two grams of industrially produced trans fats per 100 grams of fat in food.[27] Some member states, including Denmark and Austria, unilaterally set their own limits years earlier and gained public health benefits in the intervening years.

Fortunately, many food manufacturers in Western Europe have meanwhile voluntarily stopped using trans fats. But if you see "partially hydrogenated oil" on a label, the product contains trans fats. You're more likely to encounter trans fats in takeaway meals than in labelled store-bought foods, but you can't know for sure because there's no obligation for takeaway outlets to tell you what the food is fried in.

The fourth source of energy

So far, I have told the truth but not the whole truth about sources of energy. I mentioned three sources: carbohydrates, fats, and protein. There is a fourth source: alcohol. Alcoholic drinks have plenty of calories but are not recommended as a source of energy because, unlike energy-providing foods, they don't provide other nutrients. Furthermore, excess consumption can have negative effects on imbibers and bystanders. So drink responsibly — and have beer only if special gluten-free beer.

The calories in alcoholic drinks are not declared on the label, but one unit of alcohol contains 56 kcal (using the UK definition of a unit as 10 ml or 8 g). That's in addition to the calories in any other ingredients, such as sugar or fruit. The number of units in a drink depends on the serving size and the percentage of alcohol by volume in the drink. A glass of red wine typically contains 2–3 units, which gives 112–168 calories.

What about red wine, I hear you ask. Surely it's good for health and should be consumed every day? Well, I expect it will continue to be reported as being good for health one day and bad for health the next and subsequently good again but for a different reason. You decide.

Sugar-laden soft drinks

Now on to the other drink problem: sugar-laden soft drinks. Colas, sodas, energy drinks, and drinks with names ending in "–ade" fall into this category. These drinks have empty calories: lots of sugar, often in the form of high-fructose syrup, but little or no nutrition. If the label declares 25 g of sugar, that's six teaspoons. It's often more, sometimes much more. Regular consumption of such drinks leads to obesity and other health problems.

Even diet versions of soft drinks can lead to obesity because the sugar is replaced by artificial sweeteners, which fool the body into reacting as if you had eaten sugar.

Note that if the brand name of a sugar-laden, artificially flavoured soft drink is the same as one used on a mineral water, it's still bad for you — even if the packaging features a scenic view of a mountain lake or some fresh fruit.

Many people could improve their nutrition considerably just by changing their drinking habits.

Soy

Soy beans are a good source of many vitamins and minerals and some amino acids, but health claims about soy revolve around the isoflavones genistein and daidzein. Although some people (especially manufacturers of soy-based products) claim that the isoflavones have many health benefits, others (including some nutritionists) claim that they have many adverse effects. Some studies conclude that soy prevents breast cancer, whereas others conclude that it actually promotes breast cancer. There are also conflicting claims for other aspects of health.

Men should note that soy isoflavones are phytoestrogens — substances that mimic the action of the female hormone estrogen. As with other claims about soy, the evidence as to the effects of the phytoestrogens on testosterone levels in men is mixed.

Soy also contains anti-nutrients — substances that interfere with the absorption of certain other nutrients. The anti-nutrients, along with the phytoestrogens, are reduced during the long fermentation traditionally used in Asia but not in modern factory processes.[28]

Given the conflicting evidence, I cannot offer definitive advice on the consumption of soy-based products. All I can say is that I personally keep consumption of soy to a minimum, not only due to the conflicting evidence but also to be consistent with the principle of avoiding processed food; the forms of soy most commonly used in western diets, including tofu and textured vegetable protein, are highly processed. I occasionally season a dish with a little tamari and very occasionally make a miso soup, but that's all. I look for good quality tamari and miso, fermented in the traditional way. I would not take a food supplement containing soy isoflavones.

Meat glue

Meat glue is an enzyme used to glue small pieces of meat into larger chunks. Thus, something that looks like a steak could actually consist of several smaller pieces of meat.

The enzyme in meat glue is transglutaminase. If you have been diagnosed with, or tested for, celiac disease, you may recognize this name; the immune system of a celiac makes antibodies to its own tissue transglutaminase (tTG), and the presence of those antibodies in your blood is one possible indicator of celiac disease. However, there are several transglutaminase enzymes, and the tTG in humans is different from the transglutaminase in meat glue. But is it sufficiently different? Some meat glues come from the blood plasma of pigs and cattle, whereas others are produced by cultivating bacteria. The latter is called microbial transglutaminase (mTG). Germany's Institute for Risk Assessment issued an opinion paper in 2011 saying that mTG, together with food proteins, can form compounds structurally similar to gluten and that it is not known whether this affects the health of celiacs, due to insufficient clinical studies.[29]

Meat glue is legal in some countries but banned in others. It's legal in America, Canada (microbial only), Australia, and Japan. It's banned in the EU. In countries where it is legal, it may be labelled as "TG enzyme" or "TGP enzyme" and meat containing it may be labelled as "formed" or "reformed", for example, "reformed beef".

Try to avoid meat glue, even if it turns out not to be a specific health risk for celiacs. Unfortunately, this is easier said than done if you live in a country where meat glue is legal. Because meat glue is less visible when cooked, it was originally used mostly in cheap products sold or served ready-cooked, such as deli meats and hot dogs. However, meat glue is also used in steaks sold raw to restaurants and here it poses a risk of food poisoning. Normally, the part of a steak most likely to be contaminated with bacteria is the outside, due to exposure during slaughter and transport. Those bacteria are killed during cooking, even if the steak is cooked rare. But if you don't know that the restaurant is using glued meat and you order your steak rare, the cooking might not destroy the bacteria on the inside — which may consist of meat that was originally on the outside.[30] Furthermore, famous chefs now use meat glue in molecular gastronomy to create things like shrimp noodles or a surf 'n' turf dish in which the meat and fish are glued together. My advice to anyone living in a country where meat glue is allowed is (1) avoid processed meat, (2) ask restaurant staff about the provenance of their meat, and (3) avoid restaurants where the chef is a practitioner of molecular gastronomy.

When to eat

"Eat breakfast like a king, lunch like a prince, and dinner like a pauper": so said nutritionist Adelle Davis. "Skip or delay breakfast": so say many people now.

Scientific studies on the links between the timing of eating and health outcomes have given conflicting results. Research into the question "Is breakfast really the most important meal of the day?" is summarised in an article on BBC Future.[31] That article covers many confounding factors, including the following: perhaps it's not breakfast-skipping or breakfast-partaking that's a factor in weight control but rather a change of routine; perhaps breakfast-skippers have different health-related habits than others; perhaps it depends on what types of foods are in your breakfast; perhaps the timing of dinner is more important.

What to do while awaiting a definitive answer to the breakfast controversy? My personal rules are: (1) Make the overnight fast last at least twelve hours, so that the digestive system then gets a chance to finish working on partially digested food, (2) Achieve the 12-hour fast by refraining from eating late in the evening, not by delaying breakfast, and (3) Make breakfast a high-protein, low-carb meal. This suits me, but your metabolism and circadian rhythms and conditioning might differ from mine. So, experiment until you find what suits you.

Don't, however, think only of yourself. If you do plan to delay breakfast until after going to work, don't be one of those people who faint on a morning rush hour train due to low blood glucose, thus making many other people late for work. I know it happens in London, and in 2016 the Portuguese train operator Fertagus ran a campaign urging passengers to eat breakfast to reduce train delays during the morning rush hour. Breakfast-skippers, please carry some glucose tablets, so that you can quickly get some energy if you feel faint.

As for snacking between meals, it's best to minimize this unless you are very active physically. If you do snack between meals, have just one decent snack rather than grazing frequently on bite-sized snacks. If you are having a sugary snack, eating it in one go is better for dental health.

Regardless of how many meals and snacks you have, definitely try to fit all your daily eating into a period of no more than twelve hours.

How to eat

Eat slowly, taking in a moderately sized forkful or spoonful of food at a time and chewing each mouthful well before swallowing. This makes it easier for the digestive enzymes to break down the food.

Sit or stand still to eat. Don't eat on the run. Don't slouch, to avoid squashing your digestive organs.

Do not eat with your mouth open or talk with your mouth full, for two reasons. First, you may swallow air and thus get gas into your intestines. Second, it's considered rude in some cultures.

Do nothing else while eating, even between mouthfuls. If you get engrossed in a conversation or a book or in faffing about with a device, you are likely to forget to chew properly and gulp your food down. It's OK to politely inform a dining companion that you would rather eat first and then have a relaxing conversation afterward. You may even find that you enjoy your food more if you consciously focus on it while eating.

To avoid overeating, be aware of psychological factors. Following are some tips for keeping your wits about you.

- Ensure that the plates you use at home are reasonably sized. A meal served on a large plate looks smaller than actual size, and people tend to eat everything on their plates. Circular dinner plates should be no more than 25cm (10") in diameter. Side/dessert/tea plates should be no more than 20cm (8") in diameter. (Such plates are increasingly difficult to find, but you can find them by searching for "Japanese tableware".)

- When eating tapas at a restaurant where the dishes are served one or two at a time, visualize after each dish how much you have eaten so far. Although each dish is small, you could inadvertently eat more food than would fit on a dinner plate because you never see all the food on a plate at once.

- If you are female and a restaurant serves you a man-sized portion, set aside the excess food before you start eating. Ditto if you are male and you get a lion-sized portion.

- When you intend to eat a small amount from a large packet of snack food, take that amount out of the packet and put the packet away before starting to eat. That way, you won't inadvertently gobble the whole lot.

- Do not feel obliged to eat everything on a plate if you are already full. Conversely, do not feel embarrassed about getting a second helping if you are still hungry.

Meal planning

Where do you stand on meal planning? Which of the following quotations resonates with you? (1) "Life is what happens while you're busy making other plans." (2) "By failing to prepare, you are preparing to fail."

If it's the first quotation that resonates with you, you can wing it; have the principles of a healthy gluten-free diet in mind while doing the food shopping and subsequently create meals from the stuff you stashed in your kitchen.

If it's the second quotation that resonates with you, you can do detailed meal planning for a week, based on the principles of a healthy gluten-free diet, and then compile a shopping list from the plan. If you like to have a plan but don't want to keep planning, you could even use the same plan every week, in the tradition of Monty Python's Lumberjack Song: "On Wednesdays I go shopping and have buttered scones for tea".

Whether you're winging it or doing detailed planning, do revisit the "What to eat" section occasionally to check that you haven't inadvertently strayed from healthy eating. It can happen. Maybe you have to eat cold turkey every day for a week after Christmas to use it up and thus don't have any fish that week and then forget to reintroduce fish the following week, and some weeks later you realize that it's been a long time since you had any fish and wonder when and why you stopped eating it.

There are no meal plans in this book because it's unlikely that your food preferences and lifestyle would exactly match a particular set of meals. But here are some ideas to kick-start your thinking.

- Don't be constrained by conventions on which foods can be eaten at which meals. Some people think it's weird to have chicken for breakfast, though they are perfectly happy to have other meats such as bacon or sausages. Yet chicken is healthier, and strips of chicken breast can be cooked just as quickly as bacon or sausages.

- For most breakfasts, have a meal rich in protein and fat without little or no carbs. Such a breakfast makes you feel full and avoids starting the day with an insulin spike and an immediate desire for more carbs. Some possibilities are chicken or bacon with egg and avocado; a cheese omelette; salmon and cream cheese and walnuts.

- For a special weekend breakfast, make pancakes using buckwheat flour combined half-and-half with rice flour. These can be served with sweet or savoury fillings — berries or ham, for example.

- For a portable snack, put a mixture of nuts and seeds in a food bag, optionally with a few raisins or a date.

- Another good portable snack is a chunk of hard cheese, which can safely be out of the fridge for several hours in temperate climates.

- Once a week, have a vegetarian main meal or even a whole vegetarian day. Having meat or fish on most days is important nutritionally, but it's not necessary to have them every day.

- Traditional English cuisine is fine. The "meat and two veg" meal has been much maligned but that's because people used to boil everything until no taste or goodness remained. The same meal with lightly steamed vegetables is a wholly different experience. And such a meal is very suitable for a gluten-free diet because you can see exactly what the ingredients are. The full English breakfast has been similarly maligned but that's because it was traditionally a fry-up. If you grill the meat and tomatoes and poach or scramble the eggs, it is again a wholly different experience.

- For foods that are usually put on crispbreads, crackers, or toast, use rice cakes, oatcakes, or potato farls instead.

- Use leftovers. Some things actually taste better cold the next day than hot on the day of cooking. Some things are better nutritionally the next day; as previously mentioned, if cooked potatoes are chilled in the fridge overnight, some of the digestible starch is turned into more beneficial resistant starch. Furthermore, leftovers can be extremely convenient. You can put cold leftovers, such as risotto or roasted meat, into a packed lunch. Some leftovers, such as a Bolognese sauce or a ratatouille, can be re-heated to form the basis of another cooked meal. It's worth deliberately cooking extra quantities in order to have leftovers.

Rules of thumb for a balanced diet

The colour test

How colour-aware are you? In the section on phytonutrients, did you notice that the good sources of anthocyanin are all purple or blue, that lutein comes in leafy green vegetables, and that lycopene-containing foods are red? In general, if a plant food has varieties in different colours, the darker varieties contain more phytonutrients: red onions more than white onions, red apples more than green apples, purple carrots more than orange carrots, blood oranges more than regular oranges, black and red grapes more than green grapes.

Did you know that some other nutrients also tend to be associated with certain colours? For example, carotenes, which the body can convert to vitamin A, are found in orange fruits and vegetables, including carrots and sweet potatoes. (Carotenes are also found in kale and spinach, which are green because they also contain chlorophyll.) Did you know that various leafy green vegetables have several nutrients in common, including calcium, magnesium, and iron? The traditional advice to eat your greens still holds, but you also need to eat other colours.

Therefore, a rule of thumb for getting a well-balanced diet is to ensure that the food on your plate emits a variety of wavelengths on the visually perceivable part of the electromagnetic spectrum. Or, eat a rainbow and be in the pink.

The cat test

Digestion begins in the mouth, where an enzyme called salivary amylase starts the breakdown of starch. Saliva is continuously secreted, with extra being secreted during digestion. What stimulates the secretion of extra saliva? Chemicals in food, once the food is in the mouth. And the sight or smell of food, while it's still on the plate. It's good to water at the mouth before you eat because it means that digestion starts the moment you put the food in your mouth. The extent to which a food causes you to water at the mouth may indicate its quality.

If your salivary glands don't give you reliable signals about food quality, a cat could help. I was once owned by a well-trained cat, one who understood that he should eat only from his own bowl, not from his humans' plates. I would sometimes serve grilled or baked chicken breast. The chicken came sometimes from a mid-market supermarket, sometimes from an up-market one. Whenever the mid-market chicken was served, the cat took absolutely no notice. But as soon as he got a whiff of the up-market chicken, his whiskers started twitching and he became quite frantic, alternately approaching the plates because he was following his nose and backing off because he was following his training. It was obviously so difficult for him to control himself in the presence of such yummy food that I would have to cut up some chicken from my plate and put it in his bowl. I conclude that a cat knows which chicken is best. This is a valid test because I didn't let the cat see the labels, so he didn't know which chicken was being served. Admittedly, it wasn't a double-blind experiment because I, as the chicken dispenser, knew which was which. But, hey, this bit is only an anecdote about a cute cat.

The variety show

Eating a wide variety of foods increases your chances of getting a good balance of nutrients. Furthermore, variety entails eating everything in moderation, which reduces your chances of getting too much of a bad thing or even too much of a good thing.

Too much of a bad thing could be the arsenic in some varieties of rice. That's one reason why it's good to serve your main meal with rice one day, quinoa the next day, potatoes on another day, and no carbs on yet another day. Incidentally, you can reduce any arsenic in rice by rinsing it well before cooking and then cooking in lots of water. Too much of a good thing could be the selenium in Brazil nuts.

A varied diet requires varied food shopping. Don't put the same things in your physical or virtual shopping cart every week. Go to different aisles or web pages. Try foods you haven't tried before. Have you tried these?

Asparagus

Butternut squash

Cantaloupe melon

Duck

Eel, jellied (maybe only for English people in the East End or at the
  seaside)

Fennel

Goat's cheese

Halibut

Italian cheese

Juniper berries

Kale

Lime

Mint

Nutmeg

Okra

Papaya

Quinoa

126

Radicchio

Sea vegetables

Turnip

Umeboshi plum

Venison

Watercress

Xmas gluten-free pudding

Yellow zucchini (yellow courgette)

Zest (the peel of citrus fruit)

If you tend to eat the same things every week or even every day, don't delay buying different foods because you think you have to find out how to prepare and cook them first. Buy them first and then you'll have the motivation to find out what to do with them.

Also be aware that the nutrition in foods can vary depending on the soil, other growing conditions, and storage. So buy food from a variety of sources if you can.

Seasonal variation is another aid to a varied diet. When a food is in season locally, it may taste better and it may feel right; swede (rutabaga) feels solid and warming on a cold winter's day but too heavy during a summer heatwave, whereas strawberries feel nice and juicy in summer but too light in winter.

Finally, don't overeat a food because it's supposedly a "superfood" (a term for which there is no legal definition). When a foodstuff is promoted as a superfood, it sometimes transpires that the prime mover is a commercial organization that wants to shift a very large quantity of the stuff. Anyway, a large quantity of a so-called superfood in your diet inevitably takes the place of several other things you would otherwise have eaten. If you take the superfood road, the fulcrum sustaining your balanced diet crumples and you stumble into the fad farm.

Chapter 5: Lifehacks

Gluten freedom is not only about buying and eating gluten-free foods. Anyone who is on the gluten-free diet needs to master certain other practicalities of everyday living.

Being prepared

When you are out and about, always carry a gluten-free snack in your bag or pocket even if you plan to be back home in time for your next meal, in case you dilly-dally on the way and can't find your way home. Some places are gluten-free deserts, and if you get waylaid in one you could have a long wait for your next meal.

If you know for sure that you will need the snack on the same day, you can take some fresh food. If you plan to leave a snack in your bag until a day comes when you need it, take a small unopened bag of nuts or a gluten-free snack bar.

You really do need to carry a gluten-free snack with you because even the best planning can backfire. Knowing that an area where I was planning to meet someone for dinner was not well supplied with restaurants serving gluten-free meals, I checked with one restaurant in advance and received assurance that they could provide a gluten-free meal. On arrival, I found that all the customers were being ushered out the door and no-one was being let in. The manager explained that they had to close because there was no hot water due to boiler failure. If this happens to you and you are prepared, you can have a drink with your friend in a nearby bar and then eat your gluten-free snack on the train on the way home.

Eating out

Restaurants serve the same portion size for all adults and thus women subsidise men. Now, as a gluten-free person, I additionally subsidise "normal" people. For example, if I ask for a burger without the bun (having checked that the burger is gluten-free), a restaurant will happily serve it — but still charge the full price. Once you go gluten-free, the pleasure in eating out is further reduced by the fear of gluten contamination.

When reading the names or descriptions of dishes on a menu, you cannot assume that the lack of mention of wheat, rye, or barley means that they are gluten-free. Usually, menus only mention the main ingredients. If the menu does not explicitly state that a dish is gluten-free, you must ask the server. Otherwise, you will get glutened sooner or later.

Even if a dish sounds as if it must be gluten-free, you must explicitly state that you require a gluten-free meal. I learned this the hard way in my early gluten-free days. I ordered a salad on the basis of the description on the menu, which contained a list of typical salad ingredients. It came with croutons sprinkled on top. Possibly, the restaurant thought that they were providing a bonus ingredient. It wasn't a bonus to me, but it's hard to send a meal back to the kitchen on the basis of its gluten content if you don't mention that you are gluten-free when you order.

Servers are human and therefore sometimes forgetful. I once ordered an omelette in a cafe and, remembering the salad crouton experience, stated that I was gluten-free and asked for confirmation that the omelette would be gluten-free. The server said she was pretty sure it would be gluten-free and checked with the chef, who confirmed this. I went ahead and ordered the omelette and also a cup of tea. The omelette was fine. The tea came with a small wheat biscuit, perched on the teaspoon on the saucer. If it's standard practice to serve a biscuit with every cup of tea, servers may do it on auto-pilot, totally forgetting the conversation they had with the customer two minutes earlier. When this happens, you can simply ask for another spoon.

Even if the server says that a particular dish is gluten-free, I worry if they don't seem to know what they're talking about or if the food has a suspiciously glutinous texture. While I'm eating, I'm wondering if I'm getting glutened and will suffer later. I hardly ever suffer later, but the dining experience has meanwhile been marred. I am reminded of the moral of Aesop's fable "The Town Mouse and the Country Mouse": better beans and bacon in peace than cakes and ale in fear. Even allegedly gluten-free cakes and ale.

Avoid places where the servers clearly don't know the answer to your questions about special dietary needs but fail to ask the chef. And places where they answer your questions too glibly. And places where the server's command of the language being spoken is not sufficient to convince you that they understand your questions.

Be careful in any restaurant or takeaway where sauces are an integral part of every dish. The sauce may start with a stock cube containing gluten, or it may be thickened with wheat flour, or it may contain soy sauce. (All soy sauces except tamari contain wheat.) Non-saucy restaurants are better. If you go to a steak house and order steak, potatoes, and peas, you can see exactly what you're getting. Even then, you may have to ask for a steak without sauce, but at least the sauce is an optional extra and not an integral part of the dish.

Safe dishes to fall back on if there are no other gluten-free dishes on the menu are jacket potatoes and omelettes. For dessert, the safe options are Eton mess or crème brûlée. The safest places to eat are those with a totally gluten-free menu.

It's not unknown for a menu to have no gluten-free options at all. And, when there are gluten-free options, they might be not what you would have chosen. You might like the sound of the beef casserole, the seafood risotto, or the vegetable soup but end up with a jacket potato or a salad. You may have to watch other people eating delicious-looking, lovely-smelling dishes while you eat a boring meal. It's not so bad in summer, when a cool salad is welcome. But having to eat salad in winter is harsh.

Another harsh thing is that gluten-free foods in cafes are often dairy-free too. Celiacs are advised to significantly increase their intake of calcium. So when I have a slice of cake in a cafe, I want a cake made with a butter-containing sponge and a creamy or buttery topping or filling. I can see creamy toppings on all the normal cakes, but I get an undecorated cake or one with a dairy-free topping. Furthermore, if the sponge part of a dairy-free cake does not contain butter, what does it contain instead? It's worth asking.

Yet another harsh thing is that some cafes sell only pre-packed gluten-free cakes in order that that they can stack them on the same shelf as the freshly baked normal cakes and still avoid cross-contamination.

The requirement for food businesses to supply consistent oral information explains why servers sometimes seem evasive when you ask them whether a dish is gluten-free. Often, they will say only that there are no gluten-containing ingredients but it's prepared in the same kitchen as the gluten-containing dishes, in a manner as if reciting a line learned for a play. Although this could mean that they suspect contamination, it could equally mean that the chef has made every reasonable effort to avoid cross-contamination yet the servers have been instructed to always recite the same line. To find out what they mean, make eye contact, watch their body language, and listen to their tone of voice. If the premises have an open-plan layout, you can also make a judgement by observing, for example, whether the same chopping board and knife are used in the preparation of normal and gluten-free sandwiches.

The takeaway message is that you must take responsibility for finding out whether the dish you are ordering is gluten-free. You must ask the server about the food. If the server does not answer your questions adequately, you must ask them to ask the chef. If it turns out that there are no gluten-free options and they are not prepared to make anything especially for you, you must walk out or order only a drink. This is no time to be shy. Your health is more important than your desire to appear polite. If you are shy, going gluten-free may be what stimulates you to find a way to overcome it.

Now let's look at the gluten content of particular cuisines.

Pizza. Let's say you are out with a group of friends in a UK town centre where the only restaurants are branches of chains and someone suggests that you all go for a pizza. Surely it's good news that some pizza chains now offer gluten-free pizza bases? Well, I'm not so sure. Pizza isn't a healthy meal for anyone, given that it consists mainly of carbohydrate. Even if you choose a vegetable topping, all the shreds of vegetables combined probably amount to no more than one vegetable portion. Nevertheless, I tried a gluten-free pizza at a well-known pizza chain. It was very, very salty. My advice is, if you must eat in a pizzeria, order a salad.

Fish and chips. Only a tiny minority of traditional British fish 'n' chip shops and restaurants serve gluten-free fish and chips. This entails not only having gluten-free batter and gluten-free (non-flour-coated) chips but also avoiding gluten contamination. So they cannot fry your fish in oil that has been used to fry fish coated in the regular batter. A few chip shops have the batter and a separate fryer ready to go and thus can supply gluten-free meals on demand. Others require an hour's notice. Others serve gluten-free fish and chips one day a week. Some places will grill or microwave the fish instead of battering and frying it. Once you have procured some gluten-free fish and chips, don't let them put malt vinegar on it.

Indian cuisine. Poppadoms are made with chickpea flour and/or lentil flour or rice flour, but check whether they are fried in same oil as wheat-based food. Chapattis and naan bread are made from wheat flour. In many Indian dishes, a sauce is an integral part. The sauces are traditionally thickened with chickpea flour, but do check in case wheat flour has been used instead.

Thai, Japanese, Chinese, and other Asian cuisines. In principle, many dishes in Asian cuisines are naturally gluten-free. A Pad Thai, for example, is served with rice noodles rather than wheat noodles. Sushi should contain just rice, fish, and seaweed. However, the stickiness in "sticky rice" is sometimes bestowed by wheat. Also be wary of any sauce that contains soy sauce (such as teriyaki and nearly all the sauces in Chinese cuisine) because all soy sauces except tamari contain wheat. Obviously, you need to avoid tempura, which is coated in wheat batter. If you eat in a Tibetan restaurant, note that barley is a staple food in Tibetan cuisine.

Mexican cuisine. A corn tortilla should, as the name suggests, be made from corn and thus be gluten-free. Just check that they are actually corn tortillas and not wheat tortillas and that the oil they are fried in is not also used for frying wheat-based food. Burritos are made from wheat flour, but you can ask for the filling to be served in a bowl instead of in a burrito.

Desserts. Dessert menus are problematic, featuring dishes in which the base is made of pastry, biscuit, or sponge and dishes containing ingredients contaminated with gluten, such as ice cream and chocolate. The first time I ate out after going gluten-free, the only gluten-free option on the dessert menu was crème brûlée. Not having had crème brûlée for years, I thought it would make a nice change and ordered it and enjoyed it. But the next four times I ate out, it was again the only option, and it's frequently the only option. I am now so sick of crème brûlée that I would rather go without dessert. Did I just say that I would rather go without dessert? Did I, the long-time owner of a ceramic tile saying "Life is uncertain. Eat dessert first", just say that I would rather go without dessert? I did, and I mean it.

Eating at social and corporate events

The good news is that nowadays organizers of social and corporate events often state on the invitation that you can let them know if you have special dietary requirements and they will provide suitable food. The bad news is that another guest may take the food intended for you, if the all the food is laid out on a table from which guests help themselves. Someone could do this innocently, simply failing to notice the little label saying "gluten free" or failing to appreciate that the two "gluten free" portions are intended for the two people who ordered gluten-free food in advance. Here's what you do to avoid this: when someone announces that the food is ready, jump out of your chair and run to the table, elbowing others out of the way.

Travelling

Travelling abroad can be difficult not only due to language difficulties but also because the gluten-free diet is not well catered for in many parts of the world. It was previously thought that the genes linked to celiac disease are most common in Caucasian populations and rare in other populations. In fact, the prevalence of celiac disease is approximately 1% worldwide.[32] But this fact may not yet be recognized in many places.

If you are going abroad, take some gluten-free food with you (if it's legal to take the food concerned into the country). Search online for "gluten free <wherever>" before you depart. Also download and print copies of Gluten-Free Restaurant Cards (www.celiactravel.com/cards) in all the languages spoken in the countries you will visit and hand one to the server when you eat out.

Although the EU Food Information to Consumers regulation has made life easier in the UK and some other EU countries, there are some EU member states that take EU funding but don't take much notice of the regulations. When I visited one such country, I had one problem after another. Servers were stunningly ignorant about the regulations. They didn't know if there was gluten in their food and some did not even know what gluten is — and didn't seem to think it was their business to know. In one restaurant, I explained my dietary needs in English and also gave them a pre-printed card with the same message in their language, and they said that they would get gluten-free food but served food containing hidden gluten. As a result, I got glutened. At another restaurant, I followed the same procedure and was advised to order an omelette. At least when they served it on a slice of wheat bread, I could see in advance that it would be a problem if I ate it. At another restaurant, the server said I couldn't have the dessert dish I had chosen because it contained milk. So I again knew she hadn't understood the card or our conversation — but I had already eaten the main course. On the day we took a boat trip to an island, I couldn't find any gluten-free food at all and couldn't get anything to eat until arriving back on the mainland at 8pm. I have since heard that other celiacs have experienced similar problems there.

It may be easier to take a break in your own country. If you live in the UK, there are many great places on your doorstep: the Lake District, the Peak District, the Cotswolds, the Jurassic Coast, the Pembrokeshire coast, the Norfolk Broads, the South Downs, the North Downs, the New Forest, the Isles of Scilly, the Isle of Anglesey, and Bournemouth, to name a few.

Some people advocate informing a hotel or B&B in advance that you have a special dietary requirement, but I have found that advance notice sometimes makes things worse. The hotel typically responds by getting in a supply of gluten-free bread. They present it to me at the breakfast table and I feel obliged to eat it, which gives me a bad start to the day. One hotel owner made a gluten-free cake especially for me and served it as a surprise when I and my travelling companion returned mid-afternoon. It was rock hard and tasted so bad that I couldn't eat it and had to find a way to dispose of it discreetly. If I don't tell a hotel or B&B about my diet, I can simply have some of the naturally gluten-free foods from the breakfast menu (eggs, tomatoes, bacon, salmon, kippers, ham, yogurt, fruit, cheese) and just say no to any offer of toast or croissants. However, if you are planning a long stay at a hotel, especially if you plan to have dinner as well as breakfast there, it's worth giving advance notice. A good hotel can then create a special meal for you, rather than simply omitting the gluten-containing parts of a meal.

If you are travelling by air on a flight long enough for a meal to be served, definitely inform the airline in advance of your dietary requirements. You don't want to find that there's nothing you can eat when you're at cruising altitude with another six hours to go. Also carry a gluten-free snack, in case of any problem with your pre-ordered meal.

Wandering around on auto-pilot

You're walking past a cafe and someone thrusts a tray of food samples in front of you, inviting you to try one free. At the supermarket, you're passing a promotional stand for a new product and someone intercepts you, offering a free sample. You're at work and someone has brought in doughnuts to celebrate a birthday and puts one on your desk. You're at a social or business event, engrossed in conversation with friends or other delegates, and someone is circulating the room, proffering light bites.

You must have your wits about you in situations where you would previously have operated on auto-pilot. You cannot accept random offers of food. This is often a good thing because it prevents you eating unhealthy food and it prevents you eating when you're not even hungry. It may even provide an excuse for refusing something that doesn't appeal to you anyway.

Nonetheless, the need for vigilance is occasionally frustrating, like the time when I bought a jar of chutney from a stall at a food market. All the flavours were gluten-free and there was a chance to try before buying — on small pieces of wheat crackers. So I had to buy without trying, only to find later that I didn't like the flavour I had chosen.

Catering for the rest of the household

When one person in a household goes gluten-free, should everyone go gluten-free? Spouses and partners are usually supportive, especially if someone needs to be gluten-free for medical reasons. But being supportive doesn't mean that they have to go gluten-free. They can be supportive by taking care when buying food and avoiding gluten contamination in the kitchen.

There is a trade-off between convenience and expense. For example, if you are having a pasta dish for dinner, it's convenient if everyone has gluten-free pasta. Otherwise, you have to boil two pans of pasta. On the other hand, gluten-free pasta costs more than wheat pasta, so some households find that 2-pan pasta is the only affordable option.

There is also a limit to how far some "normal" people are prepared to adapt their diet. When it comes to bread, for example, some normal people prefer the taste and texture of wheat varieties and may not be willing to switch to gluten-free varieties or to give up bread.

A good compromise is to serve naturally gluten-free meals (meat and vegetables, for example), which everyone can eat, and have a supply of wheat or rye bread for the normal people. If the normal people occasionally want a meal based on gluten-containing ingredients, they can have it when eating out or they can make it themselves. That's if they still want it; if they have effectively been on a reduced-gluten diet for a while due to living with a gluten-free person, they may find that they no longer want to fill up on pizza or pies.

Getting food on prescription

If you live in the UK and have a diagnosis of celiac disease or dermatitis herpetiformis, you can get some gluten-free bread and flour mixes on NHS prescription.

Prescriptions aren't economical for everyone. They're no good if you limit your intake of gluten-free bread and pre-mixed flours due to their inadequate taste and nutrition. If you would get only one loaf of bread on prescription per month, the prescription would cost considerably more than buying the food in a shop. And you can get your preferred brand in a shop, rather than being limited to the brands available on prescription. Furthermore, you can get your food at convenient times and places, rather than having to order it in advance and make a special trip to a pharmacy to collect it. But if you eat lots of the prescribable foods or are exempt from prescription charges, a prescription may be economical for you. Whether you can make a case on health grounds is another matter.

You can select a set number of units of foods per month from the list of prescribable products. Only a limited number of suppliers have foods on the list. Those suppliers are very keen for you to select their products rather than competitors' products. Consequently, some of them offer free samples to newly diagnosed celiacs. You can get further information online or from your dietitian. If you still want food on prescription after trying the free samples, ask your doctor for a prescription form.

In practice, the availability of gluten-free foods on prescription varies by region. Some regions have departed from the national prescribing guidelines by removing some products from the list or reducing the unit allowances. I'm not sure what the "N" in NHS stands for these days. Certainly not "national" any more. Perhaps "notional"? (I'm not criticising the hardworking and dedicated clinicians who work for the NHS. I'm criticising the system.)

Abandoning food on prescription

The UK's National Institute for Health and Clinical Excellence (NICE) periodically updates its guideline on the diagnosis and management of celiac disease. Given that NICE guidelines should include an assessment of whether ways of managing a clinical condition are good value for money for the NHS, there had been speculation that prescriptions for gluten-free food would be stopped altogether. However, changes in recent years have reduced, but not eliminated, the list of prescribable food items.

But why not change the prescription system? Prescribable foods were originally introduced in the late 1960s because gluten-free bread and substitutes for other wheat products were unobtainable in food stores. Now they're widely available. Therefore, it is perfectly reasonable to re-evaluate the situation.

The current system is not cost-effective. The NHS spent £27m on gluten-free prescriptions in 2011, but much of that money was wasted.[33] For example, two gluten-free pizza bases priced at £8.95 cost the NHS £34.00 after the addition of handling and delivery charges (pizza bases having been on the list at the time). Even if you eat lots of gluten-free bread and get it cheaper on prescription than you would in a shop, you're still paying for the wastage through taxation. Yes, I know that the NHS is funded from National Insurance contributions rather than taxes, but I deem N.I. to be a tax, since no private company could get away with selling such a scheme and calling it insurance. You pay compulsory contributions all your working life with no agreement on what risks are insured and what benefits are payable if the risks materialise. Anyway, the wasted money would be better spent on hip replacement surgery for celiacs who were diagnosed too late to prevent osteoporosis or on people with more serious diseases.

Currently, the most common argument in favour of retaining prescriptions is that gluten-free food costs more than equivalent normal food and therefore celiacs need financial assistance. I question this, for several reasons.

First, not everyone on a gluten-free diet needs financial assistance. Sales of gluten-free food have increased rapidly in recent years, and a significant part of this increase is due to people following dietary fashions. Given that these people are not entitled to prescriptions, it is evident that many people can in fact afford the extra cost. (Similarly, people who are lactose intolerant or who choose to have a dairy-free diet pay the extra cost of dairy-free milk substitutes.)

Second, a gluten-free diet is expensive only if you eat a lot of substitutes for wheat-based products. The naturally gluten-free foods (meat, fish, fruit, vegetables, dairy products, nuts, and so on) are the same price for everyone.

Third, the price differential between wheat-based products and substitutes has diminished every year for the past few years (based on my own observations). This is presumably due to increased competition in the market and economies of scale in production.

Fourth, the increased expense of some items can be balanced by savings elsewhere. I find that I no longer make impulse purchases of snack foods because most of them contain gluten. I save money on lunches because I take a packed lunch to work. And I eat out less often. The net result is that my food bill is about the same as it was before.

Finally, people on low incomes who do need financial assistance would be better served by other schemes. One possibility is a voucher scheme, whereby celiacs on means-tested benefits would be given vouchers that they could spend in supermarkets. Then they could, for example, choose between having a lot of a cheap brand of bread or less of a higher quality brand. Another possibility is a system like the one in Canada, where the difference between the cost of gluten-free products and the cost of similar normal products is a tax-deductible expense.[34] Note that only the difference is paid, not the full amount. This is fairer than expecting other taxpayers to pay the full cost of something you would buy even if you weren't on a gluten-free diet.

If you can afford to buy your own food but choose to get it on prescription, don't complain if someone you know is told that they will have to wait a long time for medical treatment they need on the NHS.

Helping an illiterate celiac

If you've had to use a pre-printed restaurant card abroad because you can't read the language, you've glimpsed what it feels like to be illiterate. Anyone who needs to be gluten-free for medical reasons should read the labels on all food they buy and the allergen information on menus, but this is impossible for anyone who is functionally illiterate. If you know such a person, offer to help them with their food shopping until they know which brands of their favourite foods are allowed on the diet. Also print some Gluten-Free Restaurant Cards (www.celiactravel.com/cards) in the main language of your country for them to hand to servers in restaurants.

Going into hospital

In September 2012, the BBC reported that some British hospitals don't cater for gluten-free diets and that ward staff may be ignorant of the needs of patients with celiac disease.[35] A patient was offered toast for breakfast, given fish fingers for lunch, and had gravy and a Yorkshire pudding put onto a dinner that would otherwise have been gluten-free. When she complained about the fish fingers, she was asked why she couldn't just pick the breadcrumbs off them. The story says that the problem is being solved due to "a new policy that is now in place". Oh, yeah? Five years later, celiacs who have been in some NHS hospitals were still complaining about ignorance among hospital staff or, in cases where nurses try to be helpful, unavailability of gluten-free options (let alone healthy gluten-free options).

The BBC story says that your dietary needs are better catered for if you have a planned hospital admission rather than an emergency one and that you can ask to see a dietitian or speak to the caterers. Given all the stories about how the NHS is struggling to deliver basic healthcare, I say good luck with that and I reiterate my advice to always carry a gluten-free snack with you. If you have to stay in hospital, ask someone to bring portable, healthy, gluten-free snacks that you can use to supplement the hospital diet — fruit, raw vegetables, nuts, dark chocolate, and so on. Or even get someone to bring a complete homemade meal in a container to replace a hospital meal.

To be really healthy, try to stay out of hospital altogether. Thus you will avoid not only poor nutrition but also hospital-acquired infections, interrupted sleep, undignified experiences, and lack of natural light and fresh air.

Getting notified of product recalls

In the UK, when allergy labelling is found to be incorrect, or when there is another food allergy risk, the food product has to be withdrawn or recalled. When this happens, the FSA issues an allergy alert. You can receive alerts by email or SMS text for any or all of the 14 allergens. To subscribe, go to the following page on the FSA website: www.food.gov.uk/news-alerts/subscribe/alerts.

Other countries also provide ways to be alerted to product recalls. See the website of your food regulator.

Dobbing in an incorrectly labelled product

In most countries, the information leading to a product recall may come from consumers, producers, or inspectors. If you as a consumer believe that a "gluten-free" product actually contains gluten, or if you find that the label does not conform to applicable regulations, go to the website of the food regulator in your country for information on how to report it.

In the UK, start at the FSA's problem reporting page (www.food.gov.uk/enforcement/report-problem). Note that it suggests reporting problems to your local Trading Standards office but also links to a form provided by Citizens Advice. It turns out that Citizens Advice logs the complaints in a database accessible by all Trading Standards offices nationwide, whereas a complaint sent to your local Trading Standards office is accessible only by that office. Sometimes several complaints are needed to trigger effective action; individual complaints do not necessarily lead to immediate enforcement steps being taken. Therefore, it's better to report a problem to Citizens Advice in order to help to amass a weight of evidence.

Avoiding non-food sources of gluten

Gluten is only a problem if you ingest it, not if you anoint yourself with it or handle it. But life can be a hand-to-mouth existence. So there are a few things to be aware of regarding non-food sources of gluten.

Skincare products containing wheat are OK because any gluten remaining in the product after refinement does not penetrate the skin. For personal care products that could find their way into your mouth — facial washes, shampoos, lipsticks — look for gluten-free varieties, even though the risk of ingesting a quantity of gluten sufficient to cause a reaction is low. For products intended for oral use — toothpastes, mouth washes, floss — definitely get gluten-free varieties.

If wheat is an intentional ingredient of a personal care product, it will be in the list of ingredients. But there is no requirement for manufacturers to declare the definite presence of gluten on labels or to provide "may contain" statements. So how can you know whether your preferred toothpaste contains gluten? Most dental products are gluten-free, but formulations and production processes change occasionally. If there is no statement about gluten on the packaging or on the manufacturer's website, ask the manufacturer.

There's a widespread myth that the glue in gummed envelopes contains gluten. But the Envelope Manufacturers Association says "Remoistenable adhesives are derived from corn starch and do not contain wheat or rye gluten". So it's OK to lick envelopes.

There's also a myth that gluten is used to seal tea bags. They're actually sealed with polypropylene. So that's all right then. Except that it means they're not fully biodegradable. Loose-leaf tea is better, anyway.

Some food packaging is made from wheat straw. It is considered environmentally friendly because it is produced as a residue of food production and is biodegradable. However, packaging derived from wheat gluten can be used in containers and wrappings used for takeaway food and fresh fruit and vegetables, where it comes into direct contact with the food. Even direct contact is probably OK; some manufacturers of plant biomass materials state that their products are gluten-free or made from other plants besides wheat or derived from wheat but safe for people with wheat allergies. However, it has to be said that not much research has been done into the allergy risks of biomaterials used in food packaging.

On a more playful note, Play-Doh contains wheat and, according to the manufacturer's website, can have adverse reactions. So don't play with it, in case you accidentally transfer it from your hands to your mouth. Get your own toys instead of taking some kid's toys.

By the way, it's OK to walk by a field of wheat because there's no risk of ingesting gluten.

Eating out reprised

Ordering food at the bar in a pub. "I need to have gluten-free food. Is your fish pie gluten-free?" "Well, you'd better not have that because it's got milk in it." "But I don't need to avoid dairy products. I only need to avoid gluten." "Ah, but it's got potato too."

Questioning a server who was proffering a bread basket. "Have you got any gluten-free bread?" "I've got brown bread."

Looking at the menu, server waiting to take my order. "Do you have any gluten-free meals?" "You want a free meal?" Incredulous look. "Well, that would be nice but what I actually asked for was a gluten-free meal." Nonplussed look.

Looking at the menu, server waiting to take my order. "I need gluten-free food. Is the Pad Thai gluten-free?" "No, it contains rice noodles and I know you have to avoid rice on a gluten-free diet." "But rice is gluten-free." "I don't think so. Another customer came here a few weeks ago asking for gluten-free food and said that rice isn't gluten-free." "But it is usually gluten-free, unless it's been contaminated or the packaging says it contains gluten. Does the packaging on your rice noodles state that it contains gluten?" "I'm only going on what the other customer said."

At a burger stand at an open-air festival. "Are the burgers gluten-free?" "I don't know. I didn't ask the butcher who supplied them what's in them."

Admittedly, these incidents happened before the EU Food Information to Consumers regulation came into force in December 2014. So things like this should no longer happen. Yet in May 2015, I encountered a bed-and-breakfast hotel where the proprietor had not even heard of gluten. And in December 2015, another B&B proprietor had bought some rye bread in response to an advance request for gluten-free food. (Yes, I know I said I prefer not to give advance notice of my dietary requirements, but I sometimes do so in the name of research.) Fortunately, to give me a choice, this proprietor had also bought another loaf of bread, which was actually gluten-free — but then served it in the same bread basket as my companion's wheat bread, actually in contact with the wheat bread. Maybe she took the etymology of the word *companion* literally ("one with whom one shares bread"). Anyway, I still encounter ignorance or carelessness about gluten in food businesses.

Ordering a meal in a restaurant: "Is the beef stroganoff gluten-free?" "Yes." "Are you sure? There's no wheat flour in the sauce?" "I'll just check with the chef ... You did the right thing by asking. It's not gluten-free."

Other lifehacks

Nothing to do with gluten-free diet, but important...

- Look after your dental health: floss your teeth every day; replace your toothbrush monthly; have a dental check-up twice a year.

- Monitor your blood pressure regularly — at least once a month if it's normal or as advised by your doctor if it's high or borderline.

- Have eye tests regularly — at least once every two years if your vision is normal or as advised by your optician if you wear glasses or contact lenses or have an eye disease.

- Replace your pillow yearly to avoid over-exposure to dust mites, dead skin cells, and oil and to have adequate support for your neck. If you wash a washable pillow, tumble dry it immediately afterward and note that washing does not prevent shape-shifting so you still need to replace it within two years.

- If your shoes have laces, always double knot them to avoid tripping over them.

- Minimize multitasking. You are not as good at it as you think, even if you are female.

- If your work is sedentary, have a physical hobby. If your work is physical, have a mind-expanding hobby. If you are retired, keep active physically, mentally, and socially.

- Stop and smell the flowers, stop and listen to the birds, stop and look at the rainbow, and stop and pop the bubble wrap.

Chapter 6: What you don't need

Although you need gluten-free food, you don't need the trappings of a gluten-free diet.

You don't need a gluten-free recipe book

Why would you need a gluten-free recipe book? Many recipes are naturally gluten-free — think pork with apple sauce, coq au vin, and salmon cooked in a creamy leak sauce and served on a cot of rice. (Think "cot" rather than "bed" if you're taking on board the advice to moderate carb intake.) Yet people have spent time producing recipes such as gluten-free seafood pasta bake and gluten-free meatballs with herb salad. Well, if you want a seafood pasta bake, why not just use your usual recipe and substitute rice/corn/buckwheat pasta for the wheat pasta? As for meatballs, they should not contain grains anyway. Just add whatever seasonings you like to some minced meat and optionally bind it together with an egg. And if you want herb salad on the side, just chuck some salad vegetables and fresh herbs into a bowl and toss them in a dressing. Though why anyone would serve meatballs with salad is beyond me. Meatballs belong in a hearty winter meal, whereas salad is a cooling summer dish.

Another reason for avoiding special gluten-free recipes is that some of them are weird. Gluten-free recipes don't have to be weird. They simply have to be free of wheat, rye, and barley. Now here's the really weird thing: the ingredients in some allegedly gluten-free recipes actually feature gluten-containing ingredients, such as spelt flour or couscous. Or they are illustrated with a photo showing wheat bread as an accompaniment. So you have to pay as much attention to recipes as to the labels on processed food.

Furthermore, many special gluten-free recipes are unhealthy. It seems that most recipes for gluten-free pizza dough have sugar, maple syrup, or honey as an ingredient, whereas this is rare in regular pizza recipes. Similarly, I've seen a recipe for gluten-free salad dressing with sugar, whereas I've never seen this in a regular salad dressing recipe (which should be naturally gluten-free anyway). So if you do follow a special gluten-free recipe, don't blindly follow it. Omit unnecessary ingredients.

Often, you don't need a recipe at all. For a main course, you can just cook meat or fish and vegetables. If there's not much food in the fridge or food cupboard, you can just take out what's there and see what you can rustle up with it. If you do need recipes — if you're still learning how to cook or would like to expand your repertoire — you can start with any good cookery book for your favourite cuisine and adapt the recipes as necessary.

So you don't need a special recipe book. You just need a few tips for savoury dishes and a few tips for sweet dishes.

Savoury Tip 1: If wheat flour is included in a recipe for the purpose of thickening a sauce, use cornflour or arrowroot instead.

Savoury Tip 2: If a small amount of wheat, rye, or barley is included in a recipe gratuitously, simply omit it.

Savoury Tip 3: To make a gluten-free roux, simply substitute brown rice flour for the wheat flour.

Savoury Tip 4: If a recipe calls for stock, ensure that the stock cube or liquid is gluten-free.

Savoury Tip 5: If a recipe calls for breadcrumbs, use rice crumbs or ground almonds.

Sweet Tip 1: Take a regular recipe for cake and simply substitute brown rice flour for the wheat flour. There's no need for special gluten-free flour mixes, which typically contain potato starch and tapioca flour. They have a bad taste and texture and are less nutritious than rice flour. The reason I bake at home rather than buying processed cakes in the supermarket is to avoid potato starch and tapioca flour. What's the point of baking your own cake if you use a flour mix that makes it taste the same as a shop-bought cake? Admittedly, things baked with rice flour alone crumble more easily than things baked with a gluten-free flour mix (though brown rice

147

flour is less crumbly than white rice flour). But taste and nutrition should trump texture. And you'll soon get used to a slightly crumbly texture. You really will.

Sweet Tip 2: Don't add xanthan gum, which is in many gluten-free recipes. Although xanthan gum glues ingredients together slightly better than rice flour alone, it also imparts a gummy texture. In some people, it causes bloating or other adverse reactions. And xanthan gum incurs tax in the UK, being standard-rated for VAT even though most food is zero-rated. (For your edification, xanthan gum is a complex polysaccharide exuded by colonies of the bacterium Xanthomonas campestris, with food and industrial uses.)

Sweet Tip 3: Use recipes that don't rely heavily on flour. There are many cake recipes with relatively little flour and a high proportion of other ingredients such as ground almonds, fruit, nuts, and oats. Examples are date and walnut cake, fruit cake, banana loaf, macaroons, and flapjacks.

Sweet Tip 4: Be careful how you get the mixture in and out of the receptacle in which you bake it. Line the thing with metal foil before putting the mixture in, using enough foil to have some left above the mixture after it has risen. After baking, let the mixture cool for 15 minutes. Then lift it out in one piece using the foil. Leave the baked treat in the foil until ready to serve and then cut it into slices.

Sweet Tip 5: Pay attention to the business of the raising agent (leavener). First, procure or make a gluten-free baking powder. The raising agent in baking powder is bicarbonate of soda (baking soda). Bicarbonate of soda is alkaline and causes a mixture to rise when it reacts with an acidic ingredient and a liquid under oven temperatures. All cakes contain a liquid ingredient but not all cakes contain an acidic ingredient. That's why baking powder additionally contains an acidic ingredient. The chemical reaction between the bicarbonate of soda and the acidic ingredient starts as soon as you add the baking powder to the mixture and continues in the oven. If you delay putting the cake in the oven, the reaction may fizzle out before it gets a chance to complete. So get organized: preheat the oven, add between three-quarters of a teaspoon and one teaspoon of baking powder to the mixture as the last ingredient, mix it in, and then put the whole lot in the oven quickly. If your cake still doesn't rise much, try modifying the recipe to include an acidic ingredient such as lemon juice or honey. Or substitute natural yogurt for some of the egg, thus increasing both acidity and liquidity.

Gluten-free baking powder has a third ingredient, usually cornstarch. This replaces the wheat starch in regular baking powder. Its purpose is to keep the powder dry, ensuring that moisture in the air doesn't start the chemical reaction prematurely.

You can make your own baking powder by mixing two parts of cream of tartar (acidic) to one part of bicarbonate of soda (alkaline). If you keep these powders in their original containers and take out a small amount and mix them only when needed, there's no need to add cornstarch. If you want to make a batch of baking powder and store it until needed, add one part of cornstarch and keep it in an airtight container. The advantage of making your own baking powder is that you can be sure it has no aluminium or other undesirable ingredients.

To test whether an old baking powder still works, put one teaspoon of it in a cup of hot water and stand back. As Duke Ellington might have said, it won't do the biz if it ain't got that fizz.

If you're making cookies, you can theoretically use bicarbonate of soda as the sole raising agent because the mixture may contain just enough acidic brown sugar or cocoa powder for the small amount of rising required. Bicarbonate of soda alone is also theoretically possible for any recipe with a significant quantity of acidic ingredients. In practice, all gluten-free baked goods seem to taste better and cohere better if made with baking powder. That's the way the cookie crumbles less.

You don't need to go to a Free From show

I went to a Free From show so that you don't have to. Having perused the list of exhibitors in advance and recognized some as purveyors of stuff with all the gustatory appeal of cardboard but none of its useful functions (like protecting items to be snail-mailed), I decided to visit my local farmers' market first to get some fresh comestibles to take with me for lunch. I think that says something.

In the exhibition hall, there were free samples galore. But it's not like a normal food festival, where you can sample and buy cheese at one stand, stuffed olives at the next stand, and venison burgers round the corner. Here, it's mostly stand after stand of gluten-free substitutes for wheat-based products — in other words, a lot of processed food. Many stands were showcasing bread, crispbreads, biscuits, and cake mixes, most of which tasted like cardboard. In the name of research, I tried some brands that were new to me. Unfortunately, all that free food did not constitute what I call lunch. It turns out that there's no such thing as a free gluten-free lunch.

Notable by their absence were the best makers of pre-packed gluten-free food. Nonetheless, there were some good products at the show. But you don't have to go to such a show to find them. Most of the best products come from small companies, many of which sell only, or mainly, through online distributors. Some exhibitors weren't even selling their wares at the show or they had only a small supply of a small part of their range; they were just promoting the products and saying where to get them online. So it's better to go online than to go to a show. Also visit your local independent health food store or deli, as some small producers sell to selected independent stores.

A Free From show could be useful if you have multiple allergies or dietary restrictions, as it also showcases nut-free foods, dairy-free foods, lotions for sensitive skin, and so on. But it's no good if you have adverse reactions to children because the show attracts lots of them, many being pushed down the narrow, crowded aisles in baby buggies. I noticed too late that the advertising material included the phrase "a family day out".

Talks and cooking demonstrations were also on offer. But they were staged in an open-plan area in the middle of the noisy exhibition hall, with a constant stream of people walking past the seating area. The arrival of a restless child in the next seat before the start of a talk made me realize that there's a limit to what I am prepared to do in the name of research, especially when I've just eaten gluten-free bread. So I can't tell you whether the talks were any good.

The Free From show actually drove me to drink. I'm almost teetotal (a glass or two of Pimm's around Wimbledon time suffices for a year) yet I found myself imbibing a sample of Crop Circle gluten-free beer. I don't even like beer, but I have to say that this was just the thing to refresh the palate after eating gluten-free bread. Emboldened by that experience, I also tried a different brand of stronger beer.

After that little adventure, I realized that the sun had come out and decided that it was time to practise what I preach. So I left the show and went outside to get some naturally gluten-free vitamin D and to eat the food that my sober self had thoughtfully brought along.

You don't need teff flour

Most lists of gluten-free foods include teff. Indeed, it's listed in this book — but only because you might see teff flour in specialist stores and, given that it's flour, you might wonder whether it's gluten-free. Yes, it is. You might also wonder whether it's a suitable substitute for wheat flour. No, it's not. Apparently, it's used to make Ethiopian flat bread. Maybe it works for that (if you've got the patience to wait three days for the fermentation, as specified in recipes), but it doesn't work as a substitute for wheat in other flour-based recipes. Having bought a bag of it for research purposes, I really tried to make it work in several recipes but the results were disastrous, even when mixed with other flours. Don't let anyone sell teff to you as a gluten-free marvel.

You also don't need what teff flour epitomizes. Because teff is not widely available, you have to go to a so-called health food store to get it. Now, why are these places called health food stores, given that they sell processed food rather than fresh food and that a large proportion of their shelf space is given over to various tablets, capsules, and powders? Anyway, if you go there to get some teff flour, you will be confronted by other exotic flours and grains, which you might be tempted to buy just because it's a nice change to have such a wide choice of gluten-free goods. But some of these are of dubious value (for example, tapioca) while others are nutritious but possibly too expensive for regular use (for example, amaranth). While you're there, you might pick up a magazine or some flyers containing articles and adverts promoting other "healthy" products, which just happen to be on sale in the store. Then you're at risk of being persuaded to buy all sorts of weird stuff.

Health food stores are useful for buying quinoa, rice flour, buckwheat products, and maybe one or two other things. But regular grocery stores and supermarkets are better for most of the other things on the shopping list for a healthy gluten-free diet.

You don't need talk therapies

Although you may initially feel slightly troubled after receiving a diagnosis of celiac disease or gluten sensitivity, you will almost certainly get over those feelings within a few weeks by just getting on with life. You don't need to go to a counsellor, psychologist, psychotherapist, or any other therapist who would encourage you to talk about your disease. You don't need to find out what your disease "means" or to learn how to "own" it or to "transcend" it. It doesn't mean anything; it just is. You can no more own your disease than you can own a cat. You can't transcend it. So you'd better direct your energy toward learning how to follow a gluten-free diet with minimum fuss.

By avoiding talk therapies, you won't be such a bore to your friends. Paradoxically, many people who pay someone to listen to them still make their friends listen to endless talk about the same thing. It seems that they just have to tell someone what happened in their therapy session.

Here's another reason to avoid talk therapies: you're rarely learning anything when your mouth is moving (anon).

Having said that, some people do benefit from talk therapies. What sort of person benefits? A depressed person. A study of celiacs with depression and state anxiety found a reduction in depression and better compliance with the gluten-free diet in a group who received psychological support counselling compared to a control group.[36] However, the counselling had no effect on state anxiety (which is anxiety that occurs in reaction to a particular situation, as opposed to trait anxiety, which is a personal characteristic).

Therefore, if you are so depressed that you cannot comply with the diet, seek psychological help. But if you are just anxious, take your mind off it by getting some physical exercise, doing something you enjoy, or helping someone who is worse off than you.

(This section is about talk therapies in the context of a diagnosis of a gluten-related disorder. Obviously, if you are a war veteran suffering from post-traumatic stress disorder or you have been diagnosed with another mental disorder, get all the help available to you, including talk therapies if prescribed.)

You don't need desperate marketing

Why are so many of the organizations and companies in the special diets business so bad at marketing? I have received email newsletters worthy of inclusion in the Desperate Marketing column in *Private Eye*, making tenuous connections between gluten-free foods and things like royal family events, and worse.

Several companies and organizations in the gluten-free arena are not only desperate about marketing but incompetent at it too. Two of the companies that sent me free samples of their prescribable products made me create an account and then put my password in clear text in the confirmation email. I have more than once been automatically added to an email distribution list but not provided with an easy way to unsubscribe. I've received emails in Comic Sans font and emails that are impossible to read on a mobile device. Worst of all, I've received emails with other subscribers' email addresses in the "To" field (and thus my email address in those people's copies). If I had known all this in advance, I would have created a separate email address for dealing with gluten-free organizations; something you could consider.

Chapter 7: On the horizon

Currently, the only treatment for celiac disease is a lifelong gluten-free diet. However, the increase in the number of people diagnosed with celiac disease has not gone unnoticed by the pharmaceutical industry and scientists, so drugs are being developed and other approaches are being researched.

Drugs

Various approaches are being taken to the development of drugs for gluten-related disorders. Possibilities include a drug that breaks down gliadin (the indigestible part of gluten), a drug that binds to gliadin during its transit through the digestive system, and a vaccination that blocks the immune system reaction to gluten. The aim in all cases is that taking the drug would enable you to eat gluten without getting a reaction.

Personally, I wouldn't take drugs. I already have a treatment, the gluten-free diet. I got used to it very quickly. It works. It has no side effects. It has led me to have a healthier diet than I previously had. Why would I want to risk side effects when I already have a safe and effective treatment?

However, some celiacs are looking forward to the availability of drugs. Drugs could be useful for people whose lifestyle makes it difficult for them to stick to a gluten-free diet. They could also be taken by people who have severe reactions to accidental ingestion of gluten, just whenever they are eating out.

If you want to monitor the developments or participate in a clinical trial, search the Web for "drugs pipeline celiac".

Genetically modified wheat

Scientists are attempting to produce genetically modified wheat without gluten.[37] Wheat has a gene called DEMETER, which activates enzymes that start a chemical reaction leading to the production of gluten. One group of researchers has genetically modified wheat seeds to suppress the action of this gene to an extent that resulted in a 76.4% reduction of gluten in the seeds. Specifically, they reduced the parts of the composite gluten protein that cause the immune system reaction. This level of reduction is obviously not enough to make the wheat safe for celiacs, but the researchers believe that more work will enable them to meet this objective.

The reduction in gluten will not affect the baking properties of the wheat because the modification retains the components of gluten that make wheat suitable for baking bread. The retained components are not associated with the immune system reaction in most celiacs.

Chapter 8: Cakes and ale and the good things in life

In Shakespeare's *Twelfth Night*, Sir Toby Belch asks the party pooper Malvolio "Dost thou think, because *thou* art virtuous, there shall be no more cakes and ale?" The phrase "cakes and ale" in this context means the good things in life. On a gluten-free diet, you can have cakes and ale in this metaphorical sense and also in the literal sense because it's now possible to obtain reasonably good gluten-free cake and gluten-free ale. This is one sign that gluten-free living is getting easier.

In the 1980s, there was virtually no information or regulation about gluten, and special products and menus were very difficult to find.

By the turn of the century, allergen labelling regulations had been introduced in many countries and gluten awareness had increased. But the situation was like the schoolboy report "His improvement in handwriting has revealed his inability to spell"; the improvement in allergen information revealed the inability of many food businesses to make meals and ingredients without gluten.

Since then, the situation has improved markedly and continues to improve. In Europe, it is now possible to find out whether a food product contains gluten (or may contain gluten) just by looking at the label, eliminating the need to consult a directory or the manufacturer. It is also easier to find a restaurant offering a whole gluten-free menu in addition to the regular menu, and there are some totally gluten-free restaurants.

I said at the beginning of this book that it may take a while before all food businesses stick to both the letter and the spirit of food information law. I maintain this view because I still occasionally encounter ignorance or unhelpfulness about allergens in restaurants. However, in the UK at least, a couple of widely reported prosecutions seem to have prompted restaurant owners to take the law more seriously. In March 2017, a restaurant in Wales was fined £1,200 for serving a meal described as gluten free to a customer who then had a severe reaction. Tests found that one "gluten-free" meal had over 80 times the maximum level of gluten permitted for this claim. In May 2016, a restaurant owner in England was jailed for six years for the manslaughter of a customer who had anaphylactic shock after eating a curry containing peanuts when he had specified "no nuts". Investigation revealed that another customer with a peanut allergy had had a reaction requiring hospital treatment a few weeks earlier and that the owner knew that an ingredient he was using contained peanuts.

Such legal cases may be what prompted some restaurants to adopt a new work practice: servers may no longer take an order from a customer with a food allergy and must call the manager to take the order. Some celiacs have expressed misgivings about being treated in this way, saying that it calls unwanted attention to their medical condition from other diners. Well, I have received this treatment and experienced it as a positive thing. I did indeed have to confirm in front of other people that I have an allergy to gluten and I had to wait longer for my order to be taken, but that's surely better than risking a reaction due to miscommunication between the front of house and the kitchen. (I didn't bother to explain that celiac disease is actually an auto-immune condition rather than an allergy.)

I have also noticed a decrease in gratuitous gluten — that is, the inclusion of a gluten-containing ingredient in a dish where there is no reason for it, for example, wheat flour in a curry. I guess some restaurant owners realized that they were excluding some potential customers (or having to cook special orders for them) when they could easily exclude the gratuitous gluten instead.

Now that restaurants are taking gluten freedom more seriously, private or corporate social events can be more challenging than eating out. When you tell someone you can't eat the proffered sandwich or when you ask in advance for gluten-free food to be available at an event, reactions vary widely. Some people are really sympathetic and take time to find out what you can eat and get it right and maybe even enjoy rising to the challenge. Some people think you are a hypochondriac and reluctantly provide a limited gluten-free option. Some people accept that you need a special diet and enthusiastically try to help but get it wrong because they don't know what gluten is and it doesn't even occur to them to read the labels on any products they buy in. They may even think they're being helpful by offering you a vegetarian option, typically a high-gluten dish such as a vegetarian lasagne. Really.

That's life. It is not reasonable to expect everyone else to have comprehensive awareness of gluten. After all, you may not have comprehensive awareness of other people's medical conditions. (Do you know what to do if someone goes into a diabetic coma? If you had a house guest with an allergy to sulphites, would you know where sulphites hang out?) Nonetheless, awareness of the gluten-free diet is increasing. Many people know something about the diet because they have a friend or relative with a gluten-related disorder. I have sometimes been pleasantly surprised to find gluten-free food available and labelled as such at events where no provision for special diets was advertised in advance.

Another sign of increased awareness is that the gluten-free diet has become the target of many jokes. Go and look for them. Not all of them are repeatable here. Not all of them are sympathetic. But it helps to be able to laugh at yourself and the situations you find yourself in.

Recipes

Having said that you don't need a gluten-free recipe book, I'm providing a few recipes here because each one is worthy of special attention in its own way. None of them needs a food processor, blender, or spiralizer!

Why are there recipes for sweet dishes when I have advocated a low-sugar diet? Simply because many savoury dishes are naturally gluten-free and thus do not need modification, whereas most sweet dishes contain wheat and thus do need modification. The inclusion of sweet recipes should not be taken as a recommendation to indulge a sweet tooth. Rather, they are provided so that you can use them, or other recipes modified in a similar fashion, on special occasions or once in a blue moon (a second full moon in a calendar month — did you know?).

There are also recipes for impossible pies. These are useful on a gluten-free diet but have gone out of fashion and thus do not appear in contemporary recipe books. If you want either a savoury or sweet pie with what appears to be a pastry base, make an impossible pie. This is much easier than making gluten-free pastry and the resulting "impossible" pastry tastes better than either homemade or store-bought gluten-free pastry.

Potato farls

This recipe for potato farls is provided in case you hadn't thought of replacing "something on toast" meals with "something on farl" meals. It is inspired by Irish recipes, using rice flour instead of wheat flour.

Makes 8 farls.

4 potatoes
1 dessert spoon melted butter
¼ cup rice flour, plus a tad more for dusting

On a day when you are having boiled or mashed potatoes with dinner, cook 4 extra potatoes. After dinner, mash the potatoes with the melted butter (if not already mashed with butter). Stir in the rice flour and a tablespoon of cold water and form into dough. Turn out half the dough onto a board dusted with rice flour, roll it into a circle about 1 cm (quarter of an inch) thick and cut it into quarters. Then do the same with the other half of the dough. Refrigerate the farls overnight. In the morning, dust a frying pan or griddle with rice flour and cook the farls for 3 or 4 minutes each side or until browned.

Serve hot as part of a full English/Welsh/Scottish/Irish breakfast or an Ulster fry. Or topped with poached or scrambled egg. Or with a lightly fried mixture of prawns, chopped tomatoes, and basil. Or with canned mackerel. Or with any food typically served on toast.

Farls can be kept in the fridge for a few days or frozen.

Variations:
- Add a teaspoon of dried nutmeg.
- Use a different gluten-free flour instead of the rice flour.
- Use a mixture of swede (rutabaga) and potatoes (tastier but needs more flour and no water).
- Use a mixture of sweet potatoes and potatoes (more colourful and tasty but more prone to falling apart).

- Fry with a tiny amount of olive oil or goose fat instead of dry frying.
- Grill instead of frying.

Oat muesli

This oat muesli recipe is simply a Bircher-style muesli with gluten-free oats instead of contaminated oats. It's provided because the word "muesli" has been hijacked by food producers who supply hard, dry, bland pellets, which has resulted in decreased awareness of the original healthy recipe.

If you can tolerate oats, this muesli is great for breakfast on a day when you're going to be short of time in the morning because most of the preparation is done the previous evening. You can make bowls of this gluten-free muesli at the same time as making bowls using (cheaper) impure oats for any "normal" people in your household. Just use separate utensils and label the bowls before you put them in the fridge.

Per person:

35 g (1 oz.) gluten-free oats
Milk – enough to cover the oats
Juice of half a lemon
1 handful of almonds
1 apple (preferably a sour variety rather than a sweet one)
2 dessert spoons Greek yogurt or other natural yogurt

Put the oats and almonds into each breakfast bowl, add enough milk to cover, add the lemon juice, and stir to combine the ingredients. Cover and refrigerate overnight. In the morning, grate or finely chop the apple and mix it in. Stir in the yogurt.

Variations:
- Replace some or all of the milk with apple juice.
- Vary the proportion of oats and liquid ingredients for a thicker or thinner consistency.
- Replace the apple with blueberries, strawberries, or raspberries.

- Replace the almonds with walnuts, cashew nuts, hazelnuts, or a nut mix.

- If you are really short of time in the morning, you can chop the apple and add it to the mixture the previous evening. Better to do it in the morning to prevent oxidation, though having a substantial amount of lemon juice or apple juice in the mixture helps to prevent this. If you're using berries instead of apples, they can definitely be added the previous evening.

- For pink muesli, be rough when mixing in strawberries or raspberries.

Buckwheat porridge

Buckwheat porridge is naturally gluten-free but a recipe is provided because it has to be made in a different way from oat porridge.

If you can't tolerate oats or you just want a change from oat porridge, try this buckwheat porridge. Preparation starts the previous evening.

Serves 2.

½ cup buckwheat groats

Pinch of salt

Toppings – any combination of berries, seeds, yogurt, sultanas, maple syrup

Put the buckwheat groats into a bowl, cover with water, and soak overnight at room temperature. In the morning, rinse the groats through a sieve with fresh water. Blend the groats to a fairly smooth, milky mixture with a little more fresh water, using a pestle and mortar or some other rough utensils. Put the mixture in a saucepan with two-thirds of a cup of water and the salt. Bring to the boil, stirring continuously. Simmer for 5 minutes, stirring occasionally. Serve in bowls and add the toppings.

Impossible pie, savoury

The result of this mishmash is a pie with a pastry base, meat and/or vegetable middle, and baked cheese topping.

Serves 4.

⅓ cup brown rice flour
1½ cups milk
3 eggs
1 chicken breast, cut into small pieces
½ onion, chopped
1 cup grated cheddar cheese
130 g (5 oz.) can of sweetcorn (corn kernels), drained

Fry the chicken pieces and transfer them to absorbent kitchen paper. Lightly whisk the flour, milk, and eggs in a bowl. Stir in the chicken, onion, cheese, and corn. Grease a 25-centimetre (10-inch) dish at least 8 cm (3 inches) deep with butter. Pour the mixture into the dish. Bake at 170° C (325° F) for 1 hour or until set. Serve hot or cold.

Variations:
- Use turkey or bacon instead of chicken.
- Use shallots instead of onion.
- Use another vegetable instead of corn, chopped into small pieces.
- Use a mixture of brown rice flour and buckwheat flour.

Impossible pie, sweet

The result of this mishmash is a pie with a pastry base, egg custard middle, and coconut sponge topping.

Serves 6.

1 cup desiccated coconut
1 cup sugar
¼ cup brown rice flour
½ teaspoon gluten-free baking powder
¼ teaspoon salt
¼ cup softened butter
2 cups milk
4 eggs
A few drops of vanilla essence

Put all the ingredients in a large bowl and whisk until smooth. Grease a 25-centimetre (10-inch) pie dish at least 8 cm (3 inches) deep with butter. Pour the mixture into the dish. Bake at 180° C (350° F) for 45 minutes or until set. Serve hot or cold.

Jammy delights

This recipe for jammy delights shows how you can modify an ordinary recipe to be gluten-free; the wheat flour used in similar recipes is simply replaced with rice flour.

Makes 9 biscuits (cookies).

170 g (6 oz.) rice flour and a bit more for rolling out the dough
85 g (3 oz.) softened butter
85 g (3 oz.) sugar
1 egg
Strawberry jam

Put the flour in a bowl. Rub the butter into the flour. Stir in the sugar. Beat the egg in a separate bowl. Add the egg to the mixture and beat with a fork. With your hands, collect the mixture together and roll it out on a floured board to a sausage shape. Slice the sausage into 9 pieces and shape them into round biscuits. Place the biscuits on a baking tray. Make a small depression in the middle of each biscuit and fill with jam. Bake at 180° C (350°F) for 18 minutes or until golden.

Variations:

• Use a different jam.

• Omit the jam.

Chocolate cake

This chocolate cake recipe shows that you can make a scrumptious gluten-free cake that simply doesn't need any flour or baking powder, the texture being provided by ground almonds and chocolate. It's more time-consuming and complicated than the other recipes but excellent for a special occasion.

Serves few people, doesn't last long!

For the cake:

175 g (6 oz.) gluten-free dark chocolate

125 g (4 oz.) butter

125 g (4 oz.) sugar

200 g (7 oz.) ground almonds

4 eggs, separated

For the frosting:

75 g (3 oz.) gluten-free dark chocolate

50 g (2 oz.) butter

Melt the chocolate in a dish over a pan of simmering water, without stirring. Beat together the butter and the sugar until soft and pale. Stir in the ground almonds, egg yolks, and the melted chocolate. Whisk the egg whites until stiff and gradually fold into the chocolate mixture.

Pour the mixture into a 20 cm (8-inch) cake tin. Bake at 180° C (350° F) for 40–50 minutes. Leave to cool.

For the frosting, melt the butter with the chocolate in a saucepan, stirring until smooth. Spread the frosting over the cooled cake. Leave to set.

Resources

The following lists are very selective, based purely on personal preference and happenstance. These lists will be updated at www.sophienewtonauthor.com.

Food products

Chocolate from a local chocolatier. Among others, there are Kernow in Cornwall (www.kernowchocolate.co.uk), The Dorset Chocolate Co. in Dorset (www.dorsetchocolate.com), Temper Temper Chocolate in Kent (www.tempertemperchocolate.co.uk), Gnaw in Norfolk (www.gnawchocolate.co.uk) and Rye Chocolates (www.ryechocolates.co.uk) in East Sussex.

Chocolate from afar. If you don't have a local chocolatier, it's easier to find gluten-free chocolate in online stores than bricks and mortar ones. The Chocolate Trading Co (www.chocolatetradingco.com) has a selection of gluten-free chocolate bars and pralines, including good-quality, expensive brands suitable as gifts for the special gluten-free person in your life. It also sells non-Dutched cocoa powder.

Eat Natural snack bars. Energising and tasty bars containing various combinations of nuts, seeds, and dried fruits. Some added sugar but no other additives. A 35 g bar is good for a snack. A 50 g bar is filling enough to substitute for a meal, if necessary. Widely available in UK supermarkets and other shops. eatnatural.com

Fentimans drinks. Botanically brewed lemonade, rose lemonade, dandelion & burdock, and other soft drinks containing fermented herbal extracts. Very thirst-quenching. These drinks somehow feel healthy, though they do contain quite a lot of sugar and thus should be reserved for the occasional treat or energy boost. Available in some pubs, restaurants, supermarkets, and delis in the UK and also in some parts of Europe and North America. www.fentimans.com

Nairn's Gluten Free Oatcakes. These oatcakes can be eaten unadorned or topped with cheese, ham, nut butter, or bananas for a light meal or snack. Tastier than rice cakes and healthier than gluten-free baps. No added sugar. www.nairns-oatcakes.com

Nakd snack bars. Various energising and tasty bars, each ingredients list starting with dates and continuing with a combination of nuts and/or fruits and/or spices. No added sugar or other additives. Softer than many snack bars, making them suitable for anyone whose teeth have been weakened by celiac disease. Widely available in UK supermarkets and other shops and in some other countries. eatnakd.com

Orgran vegetable rice pasta. Good taste and texture. Useful for a tricolore pasta dish. Available in some branches of some supermarkets, some health food shops, and online sellers. www.orgran.co.uk and www.orgran.com

Rizopia brown rice pasta. Good taste and texture. Available from online sellers. www.rizopia.co.uk and www.rizopia.com

Scotti rice. Top quality risotto rice (arborio, carnaroli, and vialone nano), rice pasta, and other rice products. Sold by some Italian delis and Italian cafes with a deli counter and by some online sellers. www.risoscotti.com

Wiltshire Farm Foods ready meals. Complete frozen meals, including gluten-free meals, in three different sizes delivered throughout the UK and optionally put into your freezer. Useful for anyone who is unable to shop and cook due to limited mobility or who wants to precisely control calories. Also pureed and minced meals for those who can only eat soft food. www.wiltshirefarmfoods.com

Restaurants and cafes

Chestnuts, Alfriston. Tea rooms and bed & breakfast. Homemade cakes and scones, lunches, sandwiches, and a selection of teas and other beverages. There are always gluten-free cakes and scones (so you can have a gluten-free cream tea) and the daily "specials" menu always contains at least one gluten-free meal. Owners and staff knowledgeable about gluten-free diet and happy to cater for it. Friendly, personal service. In the lovely village of Alfriston, which is also home to my favourite bookshop, Much Ado Books. 8 High Street, Alfriston, East Sussex, BN26 5TB. Tel: 01323 870959. www.chestnutsalfriston.co.uk

River Green Cafe, Norwich. A vegetarian and vegan restaurant. The menu includes lots of gluten-free dishes, all clearly marked. Some of the dishes contain interesting combinations of foods. Also hosts a cookery school and sells "globally inspired" gluten-free ready meals. The Street, Trowse Newton, Norwich, Norfolk, NR14 8AH. Tel: 01603 622448. www.rivergreencafe.co.uk

Russell's Fish & Chips, Broadway. Gluten-free fish and chips always available; no need to give advance notice. To eat in or take away. Amazingly good quality fish restaurant for a place so far from the sea. Their homemade tartare sauce is the best I've ever tasted. Friendly service too.

20a High Street, Broadway, Worcestershire, WR12 7DT. Tel: 01386 858435. www.russellsfishandchips.co.uk

Vernon Cottage, Shanklin, Isle of Wight. Lunches, afternoon teas, and dinners, all freshly prepared with good quality ingredients. The menu has gluten-free options for every type of meal. They cater for the customer with special needs; at one meal, I wanted a dish that normally contains gluten instead of one of the gluten-free dishes and they happily modified it for me. I especially recommend the seafood dishes and the salads and the gluten-free scones. In the summer, you can eat in the lovely garden. If you plan to have your evening meal there, it's best to reserve a table because it's popular and closes early in the evening. 1 Eastcliff Road, Shanklin, Isle of Wight, PO37 6AA. Tel: 01983 865411. www.vernoncottage.co.uk

Online food stores

Healthy Supplies. Sells a good selection of gluten-free foods (but not solely gluten-free foods). Delivers to the UK and, for a higher delivery charge, worldwide. www.healthysupplies.co.uk

Real Foods. An online emporium selling a huge selection of food cupboard items, including many gluten-free items that are difficult to obtain elsewhere, and also fresh food. All foods are clearly marked with symbols to indicate their suitability for special diets, including GF for Certified Gluten Free and NG for No Gluten. Delivers to the UK and, for a higher delivery charge, worldwide. www.realfoods.co.uk

Gluten testing kit

GlutenTox Home. Can detect gluten in food to the Codex level of 20 parts per million. I tried this kit with food known to contain gluten (tested positive), food known to be gluten-free (home grown, transported from the garden to the test with my own clean hands, tested negative), and two "may contain" foods (both tested negative). The instructions are easy to follow, though they contain traces of translation from Spanish. Find it online; not providing a link due to fluctuating availability from various places.

Nutrition information

Wolfram. Answers questions about nutrition (and many other things). Start by entering "nutrition" or by going to the Food & Nutrition section and then you'll see what kinds of questions it can answer. www.wolframalpha.com

Further reading and viewing

A Greedy Man in a Hungry World: Why almost everything you thought you knew about food is wrong, by Jay Rayner, 2014. Most people in the developed world have access to a plentiful supply of the foods needed to stay healthy, whether on a normal diet or a special diet; just look at the amount of food on the shelves of a supermarket. But will all those foods still be available in years to come, in view of the growing population and environmental pressures? Given that you are interested in food consumption, you might also be interested in the sustainability of food production. If so, Jay's book is a good place to start feeding that interest. (This was written before the COVID-19 pandemic, when some supermarket shelves did actually become empty. Although that situation was due to panic buying and distribution problems rather than a lack of food supply, it does highlight the need to pay attention to all aspects of food availability at all points in the supply chain.)

That Sugar Film and/or *That Sugar Book*, directed/written by Damon Gameau, 2015. A documentary in which Damon experiments on himself under medical supervision for 60 days by consuming the equivalent of 40 teaspoons of sugar daily (an amount that many Australians consume every day) and also interviews experts on health and nutrition. The film and the book cover similar ground in different ways. Very revealing about the places where sugar is hidden and its effects on the body.

Acknowledgements

Several people helped to progress this book *a posse ad esse*.

Dr. Elizabeth Lewis, experienced food scientist and director at NutraSteward, reviewed the book from a scientific perspective. I am grateful to her for correcting some errors and omissions and for *ad hoc* chats about diet.

Dr. Lin Wylie, experienced feed scientist, was also a willing participant in *ad hoc* chats about diet.

Chris Eagles reviewed the book as a fellow celiac, though she's *ad oculos* more than that when it comes to reviewing books. I am grateful to her for offering excellent suggestions.

David Bradford, a retired writer, reviewed the book for content, structure, style, and internationalization. I am grateful to him for carrying out this task *ab ovo usque ad mala*. He and I established a working relationship when we were colleagues in the IBM publications organization. Today, he writes for a quarterly journal in which he documents the history of his ancestral home in the southern United States.

Roger Blackburn deserves extra special thanks for, *inter alia*, preparing gluten-free meals while I was busy writing about gluten-free meals, reviewing a draft, and being generally supportive and an all-round good egg.

Any remaining errors, *mea culpa*.

About the author

Sophie Newton clocked up 10,000 hours of writing and editing practice before discovering that scientists have debunked the idea that putting 10,000 hours of practice into something makes you an expert. This practice was gained mainly from technical writing in the IT software industry, including work on medical and healthcare systems. She has a degree, some certificates of achievement, and some worthless certificates of attendance.

Join Sophie's mailing list to be notified of new books and for other morsels of information, by visiting www.sophienewtonauthor.com.

The website also contains resources relating to this book, including links to the items in the References list.

Index

See also the food and drink list starting on page 17.

3-a-day campaigns, 97
5-a-day campaigns, 90
acidity in baking, 148
acrylamide, 89
additives, 115
Aesop, 130
agave syrup, 108
ageing, 73, 85
air travel, 135
ALA (alpha-linolenic acid), 68
alcohol, 116
aldehydes, 68
ale, cakes and, 17, 130, 157, *See
    also* beer
allergen labelling. *See* labelling
allergy
    alerts, 141
    to eggs, 96
    to gluten, 1, 158
    to lactose, 13, 55
    to milk protein, 98
    to wheat, 1
allicin, 88
amaranth, 151
amino acids, 59
amylase, 125
anemia
    folate or B12 deficiency, 58
    iron deficiency, 54
anthocyanin

as additive, 115
colour of, 124
in food, 76
anti-nutrients, 117
apples, 124
apricot kernels, 85
arrowroot, 147
arse
    distinguishing elbow from, 15
    flatulent, 12
arsenic, 126
artificial sweeteners, 72, 117
autoimmune diesase. *See* celiac
    diesase
auto-pilot, 136
avenin, 95
avocado, 91
bacteria
    effect of diet on, 43, 78
    in fermented foods, 107
    in yogurt, 98
baking powder, 148
balanced
    diet, 42, 126
    person, 73
bananas, 90, 104
barley
    gluten in, 5, 36
    other names for, 24
beans, 92

beer, 16, 151
berries, 91
beta-glucan, 95
bicarbonate of soda, 148
bioavailability
  of calcium in food, 55
  of nutrients in supplements, 84
birds, 15
Blazing Saddles, 12
blood pressure, 75, 145
blue moon, 160
bone health. *See* osteoporosis, calcium
bottle, water, 109
Brazil nuts, 50
bread
  replacement, 41
  white vs. brown, 44
breadcrumbs, 147
breakfast, 119, 122
breakfast cereals, 95, 112, *See also* cereals
Bron-y-Aur Stomp, 9
brown bread, 44
Brussels sprouts, 87
buckwheat
  contamination of, 24
  nutrition, 48
  porridge, 165
  portioning and preparing, 94
  uses, 50
bulgur wheat, 24

butter, 68, 101, *See also* dairy products
caffeine, 109
cakes and ale, 17, 130, 157
calcium
  as electrolyte, 75
  deficiency in celiac disease, 54
  dietary sources of, 55, 97
  supplements, 84
calories
  as energy, 59, 72
  empty, 41, 70
  expressed as kcal/kJ, 80
  in alcohol, 116
  in carbs vs. fats, 64
  in chocolate, 102
  in quinoa, rice, buckwheat, 46
cancer
  breast, 117
  link with acrylamide, 89
  link with aldehydes, 68
  lung, 84
  skin, 57
canned food, 90, 93
canola oil, 68, 100
carbohydrates
  as percentage of diet, 42, 59
  balance with fat, 63, 65
  complex, 64, 69
  in quinoa, rice, buckwheat, 46
  types of, 64
carotenoids, 76, 124
carrots, 124
cassava plant, 41

catechins, 76, 101

cats, 125, *See also* YouTube

celiac disease

and nutritional deficiencies, 53

and protein digestion, 60

antibodies, 118

asymptomatic, 11

diagnosis, 8, 13

gluten-free diet for, 1, 40

health risks, 10

intestinal damage from, 9, 38

psychological support for, 153

cellulose, 64

cereals, 5, 94

cheese, 98, *See also* dairy products

Chinese food, 132

chlorophyll, 124

chocolate, 101, 169

cholesterol

and heart disease, 62

functions of, 62

in eggs, 96

in oats, 95

chopping boards, 25, 26

cider vinegar, 107

citrus fruits, 74, 91

cocoa, 101

coconut oil, 68, 101

cod liver oil, 86

Codex standard, 28, 38

Codex wheat starch, 36, 40

coeliac disease. *See* celiac disease

coffee, 109

colecalciferol, 57

colour of food, 124

complex carbohydrates, 64, 69

contamination, gluten, 6, 24

copper, 46, 84

corn oil, 67

corn syrup, 70, 71

cornflour (cornstarch), 147, 149

cost of gluten-free food, 138

counselling, 153

couscous, 24

cream. *See* dairy products

cream of tartar, 149

crop rotation, 25

croutons, 129

cuisines

Asian, 132

Chinese, 132

English, 123, 132

Indian, 132

Italian, 80

Japanese, 107, 132

Mexican, 133

Thai, 132

cupboards, 26

cyanide, 41, 85

daidzein, 117

dairy products

and lactose intolerance, 13

calcium in, 55, 97

combining with fruit, 92, 98

free from, 131

portioning and preparing, 97
protein in, 60
dates, 90
Davis, Adelle, 119
dental health
    and chocolate intake, 103
    and sugar intake amount, 69
    and sugar intake timing, 120
    looking after, 145
depression, 78, 153
dermatitis herpetiformis, 1
desserts, 130, 133
DHA (docosahexaenoic acid),
    67, 85
diabetes (type 2)
    and good bacteria, 78
    and insulin resistance, 65
    and sugar intake, 69
    diet for, 8, 63
diagnosis
    in general, 12
    of celiac disease, 13, 53
    of gluten disorders, 8
diarrhea, 9, 75
dietary staples, 52, 94
dietitians, 8, 13
digestion
    and celiac disease symptoms,
        9
    and fibre, 77
    and prebiotics, 78
    and saliva, 125
    variations in, 12
dinner, 119

dips, 27
disaccharides, 64, 69
DNA, 59
dobbing in food products, 142
double-dipping, 25, 26
double-knotting, 145
drinks, 7, 117
drugs. See medicines
duck eggs, 96
duck fat, 68, 101
durum wheat, 24
Dutching process, 104
E numbers, 115
eating, 43, 120
eating out, 129, 133
eating out reprised, 144
eggs
    free range, 81
    portioning and preparing, 96
    protein in, 60
    vitamin D in, 56
einkorn, 24
electrolytes, 75
emmer, 24
energy-providing nutrients, 59,
    116
English food, 132
envelopes, 143
EPA (eicosapentaenoic acid),
    67, 85
Epsom salts, 56
ergocalciferol, 57
essential amino acids, 59, 60
essential fatty acids, 59, 66

etymology, 5, 144

EU rules

on advisory labelling, 32

on chocolate, vetoed, 101

on food information to

consumers, 5, 31

on gluten-free labelling, 29

exercise, 72

eye health, 76, 145

face masks, 26

Fairtrade certification, 82

FALCPA. *See* FDA rules

farina, 24

farl recipe, 161

fasso, 24

fat

as percentage of diet, 61

balance with carbs, 63, 65

body, 64

cooking, 68

in quinoa, rice, buckwheat, 46

monounsaturated, 68

polyunsaturated, 66, 68

portioning and preparing, 100

saturated, 61, 68

trans, 115

visceral, 69

fat-soluble vitamins, 74

fatty acids, 64, 66

fatty liver disease, 63

FDA rules

on advisory labelling, 35

on allergen labelling, 34

on gluten-free labelling, 30

on medicines labelling, 37

fermented food, 107, 118

fibre

in food, 46, 69

types of, 77

FIC. *See* EU rules

fish

and chips, 132

oily, 56, 67, 93

portioning and preparing, 93

protein in, 60

selenium in, 49

white, 93

flatulence, 12, 77

flavonoids, 91, 103

flaxseed oil, 68, 100

flour mixes, 147

flying, 135

folate, 46, 58

food labels, 28, *See also* labelling

food list, 15, 126

food packaging, 143

fortification

of bread with nutrients, 42

of food with B12, 59

of food with calcium, 55

of milk with vitamin D, 56

Free From, 36, 150

freekeh, 24

frozen food, 16, 89

fructo-oligosaccharide, 78

fructose

overview, 64

sources of, 69, 90

fruits, 77, 90

frying, 25, 68

FSA (Food Standards Agency), 4, 141

functional foods, 76

Gameau, Damon, 63

garlic, 88

genetic modification, 156

genistein, 117

ginger, 106

gladin, 5

glucose
from carbs, 64
from protein, 60
from sugary foods, 69
level in blood, 65, 120

glucose-fructose syrup, 71

glucosinolates, 76

glue, 5, 118

gluten
avoiding food sources of, 15, 129
avoiding non-food sources of, 142
contamination, 6, 24
detector test, 27
disorders, 1, 8
glob, 24, 27
overview, 5, 36

glutened
antidote for, 106
reaction, 11
when eating out, 129

gluten-free labelling. *See* labelling

gluten-free vs. wheat-free vs. Free From, 36

glutenin, 5

glycerol, 64

glycogen, 64

goat's milk, 98

golf, 90

goose fat, 68, 101

graham flour, 24

grapes, 124

groats, 24

hand-washing, 26

harvesting, 25

HDL cholesterol, 62

health claims, 85

health food stores, 151

helping others, 140, 153

herbs, 105, 106

herring, 93

holidays, 134

honey, 108

Hordeum vulgare, 24

horsemeat, 112

hospital food, 140

hotels, 135

housemates, 26, 136

hybrids, 24

hydrogenated oil, 82, 116

illiteracy, 140

impossible pie recipe, 166, 167

Indian food, 132

inflammation, 67, 78

ingredients lists, 71, 81, *See also* labelling

insoluble fibre, 77

insulin, 65

international standards
   on additive numbering, 115
   on gluten-free labelling, 28

intolerance. *See* allergy

inulin, 78

iron
   deficiency in celiac disease, 54
   dietary sources of, 54
   in oats, 95
   in quinoa, rice, buckwheat, 46
   supplements, 54

isoflavones, 117

Italian food, 39, 80

jammy delights recipe, 168

Japanese
   food, 107, 132
   poetry, 33
   tableware, 121

kale, 55

Kamut, 24

kefir, 108

Kendrick, Malcolm, 61

kidney stones, 84

kimchi, 107

kitchens, 24

labelling
   advisory/voluntary in EU, 32
   advisory/voluntary in US, 35
   advisory/voluntary
      internationally, 35

for medicines, 37

for normal foods, 30, 79

for special dietary foods, 28

infringements, 142, 157

international standard on, 28

of health claims, 85

of sugars, 70

rants about, 32, 34

lactase, 13

lactose
   in milk, 64
   intolerance, 13, 55

language, 32, 134

lard, 68, 101

LDL cholesterol, 62

leather cleaning, 90

leavener, 148

leftovers, 124

legumes, 60, 92

lemon, 106, 115

lime, 106

linseed. *See* flaxseed

liver
   and cholesterol circulation, 62
   and glucose metabolism, 64
   and vitamin storage, 58, 74
   fatty disease of, 63

low-fat foods, 66

Lumberjack Song, 122

lunch, 119

lutein, 76, 124

lycopene, 76, 124

lysine, 60

mackerel, 93
macronutrients, 59
magnesium
 and calcium, 56
 and vitamin D, 58
 as electrolyte, 75
 in bananas, 90
 in nuts and seeds, 99
 in oats, 95
 in olives, 91
 in quinoa, rice, buckwheat, 46
 in tap water, 108
 in vegetables, 87, 124
Maillard reaction, 89
malt vinegar, 107
manganese, 46
maple syrup, 108
marketing messages, 81, 153
may contain
 EU rules on, 32
 FDA rules on, 35
 study on, 35
meal planning, 122
meat
 and two veg, 123
 glue, 118
 iron in, 54
 portioning and preparing, 92
 protein in, 60
 selenium in, 49
medicines
 gluten in, 7, 37
 herbal, 105
 interaction with food, 86

intreraction with
 supplements, 84
 on the horizon, 155
melatonin, 104
metabolism, 65
methionine, 60
Mexican food, 133
microbiome, 78
micronutrients, 74
milk, 98, 104, *See also* dairy
 products
milling, 25
minerals, 45, 75
mint, 106
miso, 118
mock meats, 24
mograbieh, 24
molecular gastronomy, 119
monosaccharides, 64, 69
monounsaturated fat, 68
Mouldy Old Dough, 20
mountaineering, 90
MSC (Marine Stewardship
 Council), 94
mTG (microbial
 transglutaminase), 118
muesli recipe, 163
multitasking, 145
muscles, 64
NHS, 137, 141
niacin, 46
Nobel Prize, 104
normal people, 26, 136
nutrition, 41, 126

nutrition declarations, 70, 79

nutritionists, 8

nuts, 99

oats

   Codex rules for labelling of, 29

   contamination of, 20, 24

   EU rules for labelling of, 29

   in muesli recipe, 163

   portioning and preparing, 94

   US rules for labelling of, 30

obesity, 63, 78

oils

   algal, 67

   contamination in frying, 25, 27

   cooking, 68

   Omega, 67, 97

   portioning and preparing, 100

oily fish

   Omega oils in, 67

   types of, 93

   vitamin D in, 56

olive oil

   cooking with, 100

   fats in, 68, 80

olives, 91

Omega oil

   in algae, 67

   in eggs, 97

   in fish, 67

   ratios, 63, 66

   supplements, 85

omelette, 130

onions, 88, 124

oranges, 124

osteoporosis

   balancing exercises for, 73

   calcium and vitamin D for, 56

   risk from celiac disease, 10, 54

overeating, 72, 121

oxidation, 100

palm oil, 67

pantothenic acid, 47

parts per million (of gluten in food), 28, 38

pasteurization, 107

pastry, 6, 160

peas, 92

peel, 91

peptides, 60

phosphorous, 46

phytic acid, 99

phytonutrients, 75, 124

pillows, 145

Pimm's, 151

pizza

   in diet, 53

   in restaurants, 132

   recipes, 146

plant foods

   iron in, 54

   Omega oil in, 68

   phytonutrients in, 75

plate sizes, 121

polyols, 64

polyphenols, 76, 104
polyunsaturated fat
  and aldehydes, 68
  types of, 63, 66
portion sizes, 121
potassium
  as electrolyte, 75
  in food, 46, 90
potatoes
  as dietary staple, 52
  as safe option, 130
  farling, 161
  preserving the nutrients of,
    88
prebiotics, 78, 107
prescriptions, 137
probiotics, 78, 107
processed food
  acrylamide in, 89
  and legume digestibility, 92
  fructose in, 70
  gluten in, 6
  gluten removed from, 16, 28
  in stores, 151
  inulin in, 78
  nitrates and nitrites in, 93
  problems with, 112, 118
  salt in, 106
product recalls, 141
protein
  functions of, 59, 66
  in quinoa, rice, buckwheat, 46
pseudo-cereals, 7, 94
pyridoxine, 46

quinoa
  nutrition, 46
  portioning and preparing, 94
  uses, 50
raising agent, 148
raisins, 90
rapeseed oil, 68, 100
raw food, 88, 93
RDA (recommended daily
  amount), 79
RDI (reference intake), 79
recalls of food products, 141
recipes, 146, 160
recommended amounts, 79
reformed meat, 118
resistant starch, 89, 90
resources, 170
Restaurant Cards, 134, 140
restaurants, 25, 129
retirement, 145
riboflavin, 46, 115
rice
  arsenic in, 126
  flour, 147
  nutrition, 47
  portioning and preparing, 94
  uses, 50
  vinegar, 107
  white vs. brown, 52
roasting, 68
rye
  gluten in, 5, 36
  other names for, 24
saliva, 125

salmon, 93

salmonella, 96

salt

  in cheese, 98

  labelling, 79

  portioning, 106

sandwiches, 43, 51

sardines, 55, 93

saturated fat

  cooking in, 68

  dietary guidelines on, 61

  in chocolate, 102

  in milk, 98

sauces, 130, 147

sauerkraut, 107

seasonal foods, 127

Secale cereale, 24

seeds, 99

seitan, 24

selenium

  in fish, 93

  in quinoa, rice, buckwheat, 47

  overview, 48

semolina, 24

serotonin, 104

sesame oil, 100

Shakespeare, 157, 172

shampoo, 142

sheep's milk, 98

shellfish, 49, 93

shopping

  for balanced diet, 126, 152

  for gluten avoidance, 28, 36

  on Wednesdays, 122

skincare products, 142

skins of fruit and veg, 77

sleep, 104

smoothies, 90

snacks

  carrying, 128, 141

  nutty, 123

  vegetable, 88

soaking nuts, 99

sodium, 75, 106

soil, nutrients in, 49, 127

soluble fibre, 77

sorbitol, 64

soy, 67, 117

spelt, 24

spices, 105, 113

spinach, 55

stanols, 76

staple foods, 52, 94

starch, 69

  in complex carbs, 64

  in gluten-free bread, 41

  resistant, 89, 90

  tapioca, 41

  wheat, 40

statins, 62

steatorrhea, 9

sterols, 76

stock cubes, 147

sucrose, 64, 69

sugar

  added/free, 69, 70

  daily limit, 69

  hidden, 70

in chocolate, 102
in drinks, 117
naturally occurring, 69, 70
other names for, 71
study on, 63
types of, 64
withdrawal, 71
sultanas, 90
summary of diet, 110
sunflower oil, 67, 68
sunlight and vitamin D, 57, 62
superfoods, 127
supplements
  Omega oil, 85
  vitamin and mineral, 53, 83
  vitamin D, 57, 84
sustainability, 94, 174
sweeteners, 72, 117
talk therapies, 152
tamari, 118, 130
tannins, 54
tapas, 121
tapioca starch, 41
tax, 140, 148
tea
  bags, 143
  effect on iron absorption, 54
  green, 103
  portioning, 109
teff, 151
testing for gluten, 27
textured vegetable protein, 118
Thai food, 132
theobromine, 103

thiamin, 46
time of eating, 119, 120
tinned food. *See* canned food
toasters, 27
tofu, 118
tomatoes, 76, 88
toys, 143
traffic lights, 80
trans fats, 115
transglutaminase, 118
travel, 134
triglycerides, 64
Triticale, 24
Triticum, 24
trout, 93
tryptophan, 104
tTG (tissue transglutaminase), 118
tuna, 93
US rules. *See* FDA rules
vacations, 134
vegan, 8, 59
vegetables
  colour of, 124
  effect on gut bacteria, 43
  fibre in, 77
  portioning and preparing, 87
vegetarian, 8, 60
villi, 38
vinegar, 107
vitamin A
  colour of, 124
  in food, 74, 98
  in supplements, 84

vitamin B, 74, 83

vitamin B1 (thiamin), 46

vitamin B12, 58, 92

vitamin B2 (riboflavin), 46, 115

vitamin B3 (niacin), 46

vitamin B5 (pantothenic acid), 47

vitamin B6 (pyridoxine), 46, 90

vitamin C

additive, 115

and iron absorption, 54

preserving in citrus fruits, 91

sources, 74

vitamin D

and magnesium, 58

overview, 56, 74

synthesis in body, 62

vitamin E, 74, 84

vitamin K

in bananas, 90

in buckwheat, 48

storage in liver, 74

vitamins, 45, 74

walnut oil, 100

Warfarin, 86

water, 108, 117

water-soluble vitamins, 74

weight change, 10, 72

wheat

allergy, 1

fields, 143

genetically modified, 156

gluten in, 5, 36

growing and trading, 5, 49

in food packaging, 143

in personal care products, 142

in toys, 143

nutrition, 45

other names for, 24

starch in, 40

uses, 50

white bread, 44

wine, 116

xanthan gum, 148

xylitol, 64

yogurt, 78, 98, *See also* dairy products

zinc

in food, 46, 92

in supplements, 84

References

[1] "Codex standard": Codex standard for foods for special dietary use for persons intolerant to gluten. Codex Standard 118. 2015 amendment. Codex Alimentarius Commission. Available at: http://www.fao.org/fao-who-codexalimentarius.

[2] "EU regulation about gluten-free foods": Commission Implementing Regulation (EU) No 828/2014 of 30 July 2014 on the requirements for the provision of information to consumers on the absence or reduced presence of gluten in food. *Official Journal of the European Union*, 31.7.2014 L 228/5. CELEX number: 32014R0828. Available at: http://eur-lex.europa.eu/homepage.html.

[3] "US Food and Drug Administration (FDA) rule": FDA, 2016. *Questions and Answers: Gluten-Free Food Labeling Final Rule*. Available at: http://www.fda.gov/food/guidanceregulation/guidancedocumentsregulatoryinformation/allergens/ucm362880.htm, accessed 04 March 2020.

[4] "EU regulation on the provision of food information to consumers": Regulation (EU) No 1169/2011 of the European Parliament and of the Council of 25 October 2011 on the provision of food information to consumers. *Official Journal of the European Union*, 22.11.2011 L 304/18. CELEX number: 32011R1169. Available at: http://eur-lex.europa.eu/homepage.html.

[5] "US legislation on allergen information": FDA, 2016. *Food Allergen Labeling and Consumer Protection Act of 2004*. Available at: www.fda.gov/Food/GuidanceRegulation/GuidanceDocumentsRegulatoryInformation/Allergens/ucm106187.htm, accessed 04 March 2020.

[6] "a UK study analyzed allergen labelling and allergen content": B. Hirst, Reading Scientific Services Ltd, commissioned by the Food Standards Agency, 2014. *Final report: survey of allergen advisory labelling and allergen content of UK retail pre-packed processed foods*. Available at: https://www.food.gov.uk/research/food-allergy-and-intolerance-research/survey-of-allergen-labelling-and-allergen-content-of-processed-foods, accessed 04 March 2020.

[7] "similar studies in the US": T. Thompson, T.B. Lyons, A. Jones., *European Journal of Clinical Nutrition*, 2016, 70:1341–47. Allergen advisory statements for wheat: do they help US consumers with celiac disease make safe food choices? doi:10.1038/ejcn.2016.155. Available by subscription at www.nature.com/articles/ejcn2016155, press release summary available at https://www.glutenfreewatchdog.org/news/wp-content/uploads/2016/09/EJCNAASPressReleaseSept15-1.pdf.

[8] "draft guidance on gluten labelling for oral drug products": FDA, December 2017. *Gluten in Drug Products and Associated Labeling Recommendations*. Available at: https://www.fda.gov/Drugs/ResourcesForYou/Consumers/BuyingUsi ngMedicineSafely/EnsuringSafeUseofMedicine/ucm410373.htm, accessed 04 June 2019.

[9] "established 20 ppm as the safe level": C. Catassi, E. Fabiani, G. Iacono, et al., *The American Journal of Clinical Nutrition*, 2007, 85:160–6. A prospective, double-blind, placebo-controlled trial to establish a safe gluten threshold for patients with celiac disease. Available at: http://ajcn.nutrition.org/content/85/1/160.long.

[10] "study published in 2013 examined the risk … of intestinal damage": A. Gilbert, A.G. Kruizinga, S. Neuhold, et al., *The American Journal of Clinical Nutrition*, 2013, 97:109–16. Might gluten trace in wheat substitutes pose a risk in patients with celiac disease? A population-based probabilistic approach to risk estimation. Available at: http://ajcn.nutrition.org/content/97/1/109.long.

[11] "good bacteria decreased and bad bacteria increased": Y. Sanz, *Gut Microbes*, 2010, May–Jun 1(3):135–137. Effects of a gluten-free diet on gut microbiota and immune function in healthy adult humans. doi:10.4161/gmic.1.3.11868. Available at: http://www.ncbi.nlm.nih.gov/pmc/articles/PMC3023594.

[12] "balanced diet must include many more vegetables": I. B. Jeffery and P.W. O'Toole, *Nutrients*, 2013, 5(1):234–252. Diet-Microbiota Interactions and Their Implications for Healthy Living.

doi:10.3390/nu5010234. Available at: http://www.mdpi.com/2072-6643/5/1/234/htm.

[13] "usage in bread-making of wheat imported from North America": C.C. Johnson, F.M. Fordyce and M.P. Rayman, *Proceedings of the Nutrition Society*, 2010, 69(1):119-132. Symposium on 'Geographical and geological influences on nutrition' Factors controlling the distribution of selenium in the environment and their impact on health and nutrition, doi:10.1017/S0029665109991807. Abstract available via the doi at www.cambridge.org/core/journals.

[14] "vitamin D levels increased in all three groups by roughly the same amount": The big vitamin D experiment. *Trust Me, I'm a Doctor, series 2, episode 1*. Broadcast on BBC Two TV on 15 October 2014. Summary available at: http://www.bbc.co.uk/programmes/articles/4mbCTBjhnt8VLmMKw Qz3RrS/the-big-vitamin-d-experiment, accessed 04 March 2020.

[15] "Dietary advice … should not have been introduced": Z. Harcombe, J.S. Baker, S.M. Cooper et al., *Open Heart*, 2015, 2(1). Evidence from randomised controlled trials did not support the introduction of dietary fat guidelines in 1977 and 1983: a systematic review and meta-analysis.: doi:10.1136/openhrt-2014-000196. Available at: http://openheart.bmj.com/content/2/1/e000196.full.

[16] "doubts had been building up for some years": M. Kendrick, *The Cholesterol Con: The Truth about What Really Causes Heart Disease and How to Avoid It*, John Blake Publishing Ltd., London, 2008.

[17] "paralleling an increase in the incidence of obesity and diabetes": J.J. DiNicolantonio, *Open Heart*, 2014; 1(1). The cardiometabolic consequences of replacing saturated fats with carbohydrates or Omega-6 polyunsaturated fats: Do the dietary guidelines have it wrong? doi:10.1136/openhrt-2013-000032. Available at: http://openheart.bmj.com/content/1/1/e000032.full.

[18] "When … oils high in polyunsaturated fat are heated, they oxidize": Which oils are best to cook with? *Trust Me, I'm a Doctor, series 3, episode 3*. Broadcast on BBC Two TV on 29 July 2015. Summary available

at:
http://www.bbc.co.uk/programmes/articles/3t902pqt3C7nGN99hVRF
c1y/which-oils-are-best-to-cook-with, accessed 04 March 2020.

[19] "WHO recommends reducing the intake of free sugars": World Health Organization, 2015. *Guideline: Sugars intake for adults and children.* Available at:
https://www.who.int/nutrition/publications/guidelines/sugars_intake/en/.

[20] "supplementing with vitamins A or E increases the risk of early death": BBC News, 28 February 2007. *Vitamins 'could shorten lifespan'.* Available at: http://news.bbc.co.uk/1/hi/health/6399773.stm.

[21] "supplementing with vitamin E increases the risk of lung cancer": BBC News, 29 February 2008. *Vitamin E linked to lung cancer.* Available at: http://news.bbc.co.uk/1/hi/health/7271189.stm.

[22] "supplementation with calcium is linked to a greater risk of kidney stones": National Institutes of Health Office of Dietary Supplements. *Calcium Dietary Supplement Fact Sheet.* Available at:
https://ods.od.nih.gov/factsheets/Calcium-Consumer/, accessed 04 March 2020.

[23] "supplementation with calcium … and plaque buildup in arteries": Johns Hopkins Medicine, 11 October 2016. *Calcium Supplements may Damage the Heart.* Available at:
http://www.hopkinsmedicine.org/news/media/releases/calcium_supplements_may_damage_the_heart, accessed 04 March 2020.

[24] "systematic review of earlier studies on oats and celiac disease": K. Garsed and B.B. Scott, *Scandinavian Journal of Gastroenterology*, 2007, 42(2):171–178. Can oats be taken in a gluten-free diet? A systematic review. doi:10.1080/00365520600863944. Abstract available at: http://informahealthcare.com/doi/abs/10.1080/00365520600863944.

[25] "nutrient analysis … chicken eggs": Department of Health, 2013. *Nutrient Analysis of Eggs.* Available at:
https://www.gov.uk/government/publications/nutrient-analysis-of-eggs, accessed 04 March 2020.

26 "nutritional points about the consumption of dairy products": Dairy All-Party Parliamentary Group, 2016. *Putting Dairy Back on the Daily Menu.* Available at: https://researchbriefings.parliament.uk/ResearchBriefing/Summary/CBP-7564.

27 "EU has set a limit… trans fats": Commission Regulation (EU) No 2019/649 of 24 April 2019 amending Annex III to Regulation (EC) No 1925/2006 of the European Parliament and of the Council as regards trans fat, other than trans fat naturally occurring in fat of animal origin. *Official Journal of the European Union,* L 110. CELEX number: 32019R0649. Available at: http://eur-lex.europa.eu/homepage.html.

28 "anti-nutrients … are reduced … but not in modern factory processes": F. Lawrence, *The Guardian,* 25 July 2006. Should we worry about soya in our food? Available at: http://www.theguardian.com/news/2006/jul/25/food.foodanddrink, accessed 04 March 2020.

29 "not known whether this affects the health of celiacs": Bundesinstitut für Risikobewertung, 2011. *Transglutaminase in Meat Products: Updated BfR opinion No. 052/2011.* Available at: http://www.bfr.bund.de/en/publication/bfr_opinions_2011-127797.html, accessed 04 March 2020.

30 "cooking might not destroy the bacteria": WTAE-TV Pittsburgh, 2012. *Is your prime steak held together by 'Meat Glue'?* Available at: https://www.youtube.com/watch?v=4PE9rdmvIz0, accessed 04 March 2020.

31 "breakfast… an article on BBC Future": J. Brown, BBC Future, 29 November 2018. *Is breakfast really the most important meal of the day?* Available at: http://www.bbc.com/future/story/20181126-is-breakfast-good-for-your-health, accessed 04 March 2020.

32 "the prevalence of celiac disease is approximately 1% worldwide": C. Catassi and A. Fasano, *Current Opinion in Gastroenterology,* 2008, 24:687–691. Celiac disease. doi:10.1097/MOG.0b013e32830edc1e. Abstract

available at http://journals.lww.com/co-gastroenterology/Abstract/2008/11000/Celiac_disease.7.aspx.

33 "NHS spent £27m on gluten-free prescriptions in 2011": L. MacKean, BBC News, 24 May 2012. *NHS 'paid £17 for gluten-free pizza base'*. Available at: http://www.bbc.co.uk/news/health-17755552, accessed 04 March 2020.

34 "a tax-deductible expense": Canada Revenue Agency, 2016. *Gluten-free products*. Available at: https://www.canada.ca/en/revenue-agency/services/tax/individuals/topics/about-your-tax-return/tax-return/completing-a-tax-return/deductions-credits-expenses/lines-330-331-eligible-medical-expenses-you-claim-on-your-tax-return/details-medical-expenses.html, accessed 04 March 2020.

35 "some British hospitals don't cater for gluten-free diets": BBC News, 2012. *Do hospitals cater for patients with special diets?* Available at: http://www.bbc.co.uk/news/health-19763163, accessed 04 March 2020.

36 "celiacs with depression and state anxiety": G. Addolorato, G. De Lorenzi, L. Abenavoli, et al., *Alimentary Pharmacology & Therapeutics*, 2004, 20: 777–782. Psychological support counselling improves gluten-free diet compliance in coeliac patients with affective disorders. doi:10.1111/j.1365-2036.2004.02193.x. Available at: http://onlinelibrary.wiley.com/doi/10.1111/j.1365-2036.2004.02193.x/full.

37 "genetically modified wheat without gluten". W. Shanshan, W. Nuan, J. Pang et al., *Proceedings of the National Academy of Sciences of the United States of America*, 2012, 109(50):20543–20548. Structural genes of wheat and barley 5-methylcytosine DNA glycosylases and their potential applications for human health. doi:10.1073/pnas.1217927109. Available at: http://www.pnas.org/content/109/50/20543.full.